T0110371

Praise for *The Meaning of Sunglasses*:

"[An] uproarious dictionary of style (or what passes for it)."
—*The New York Times*

"Wildly entertaining."   —*Entertainment Weekly*

"A cute, zippy, and often hilarious little book about fashion."
—Teen Vogue.com

"If you want to know what makes the fashion world go round, read *The Meaning of Sunglasses*. Good fashion writers with a clear, clever voice are rare and wonderful things and Hadley Freeman is one of them."   —*The Observer* (London)

"Here is a wry book that will make enjoyable reading for anyone wondering how best to clothe themselves for this new century. Refreshingly down-to-earth and witty; I found myself laughing aloud."   —*The Guardian* (London)

"Here is both a sensible and funny guide to fashion. This book is informative and amusing."   —*Deseret Morning News*

"Lighthearted and all-inclusive, Hadley Freeman decodes the language known as 'fashionspeak.'"   —*The Daily Texan*

PENGUIN BOOKS

THE MEANING OF SUNGLASSES

Hadley Freeman is the deputy fashion editor of *The Guardian*, where she writes the popular column "Ask Hadley." Freeman attended Oxford University and received the Catherine Pakenham journalism prize. She is a contributing editor for British *Vogue* and lives in London.

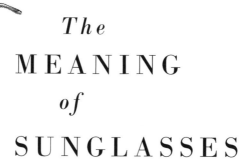

The

MEANING

of

SUNGLASSES

✧

And a Guide to Almost All Things Fashionable

HADLEY FREEMAN

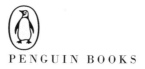

PENGUIN BOOKS

PENGUIN BOOKS

Published by the Penguin Group

Penguin Group (USA) Inc., 375 Hudson Street, New York, New York 10014, U.S.A.
Penguin Group (Canada), 90 Eglinton Avenue East, Suite 700, Toronto, Ontario, Canada
M4P 2Y3 (a division of Pearson Penguin Canada Inc.) • Penguin Books Ltd, 80 Strand,
London WC2R 0RL, England • Penguin Ireland, 25 St Stephen's Green, Dublin 2, Ireland
(a division of Penguin Books Ltd) • Penguin Group (Australia), 250 Camberwell Road,
Camberwell, Victoria 3124, Australia (a division of Pearson Australia Group Pty Ltd) •
Penguin Books India Pvt Ltd, 11 Community Centre, Panchsheel Park, New Delhi – 110
017, India • Penguin Group (NZ), 67 Apollo Drive, Rosedale, North Shore 0632, New
Zealand (a division of Pearson New Zealand Ltd) • Penguin Books (South Africa) (Pty) Ltd,
24 Sturdee Avenue, Rosebank, Johannesburg 2196, South Africa

Penguin Books Ltd, Registered Offices:
80 Strand, London WC2R 0RL, England

First published in the United States of America by Viking Penguin,
a member of Penguin Group (USA) Inc. 2008
Published in Penguin Books 2009

Illustrations by Gina Adams

THE LIBRARY OF CONGRESS HAS CATALOGED THE HARDCOVER EDITION AS FOLLOWS:
Freeman, Hadley.
The meaning of sunglasses : and a guide to almost all things fashionable / by
Hadley Freeman.
    p.   cm.
ISBN 978-0-670-01867-3 (hc.)
ISBN 978-0-14-311499-4 (pbk.)
1. Sunglasses. 2. Fashion. I. Title.
GT2370.F74 2008
391.4—dc22   2007027532

146122990

For my mother and father,
who taught me that i *goes before* e *and how to wear shorts*

Contents

Acknowledgments

So many people to thank, so little desire to inflict a load of mwah-mwah acknowledgments on the reader. Oh, well, tough luck. And so, a big thank-you to:

Ian Katz for everything; Katharine Viner and Merope Mills for maintaining a sorely tested belief that there might be some wheat despite all the chaff; Jess Cartner-Morley for being the best editor, inspiration, and friend a lady could ever hope to find; Alexandra Shulman for endlessly appreciated support and encouragement; the two Kates in my life, Jones and Barker, the supersonic agent and editor, and their respective entourages—Laura Sampson at ICM and Venetia Butterfield, Tom Weldon, Eleo Gordon, and John Hamilton at Viking; Heather Schroder at ICM and Hilary Redmon at Penguin for nobly flying the American flag; Imogen Fox, Priscilla Kwateng, Stevie Brown, Paula Cocozza, Kathy Chan, and honorary fashion-desk members Ben Clissitt and Simon Chilvers for personal styling and personal therapy; Sophia Neophitou, Antony Miles, and Dan May for never telling me to shut up; my family for never doubting the veracity of my opinions in spite of all evidence to the contrary; and Carol Miller, Charlie Porter, the Ibizans, Marina Hyde, Simon Woods, Jamie Dornan, Poppy de Villeneuve, Conrad Shawcross, Sally Henderson, Myles Macinnes, Catherine Boyd, Helen Seamons, Patrick Kennedy, Martin Tisne, and Tessa Bilder for always ensuring I get home safely at the end of the night. You're all fabulous. Mwah.

Introduction

In one characteristically if particularly prescient episode of the TV show *South Park*, originally aired all the way back in 2004, Paris Hilton came to the animated eponymous town in Colorado to open a store, marketing her distinctive look to the mountain-bound eight-year-old girls. Now, leaving aside the aesthetic merits or otherwise of this concept, her appearance raised an interesting question: is it, as one character claimed, "empowering" to encourage girls and women to dress in a particular style, or does it, as another stoutly put it, turn you into a "stupid, spoiled . . ." and there, for decency's sake, we must abruptly stop quoting from *South Park*, but you probably get the idea.

Of course, the question as it relates specifically to dressing like Hilton is fairly easy to resolve, but, in regard to fashion as a whole, it is, judging by the arguments exercised by some with the kind of tirelessness that would impress a Russian Olympic athlete, more complicated. Is fashion one big, nasty, anachronistic, and misogynistic conspiracy to make women feel inadequate, or is it a means for self-expression that actually brings a lot of gratification?

If one were to go just by the way fashion tends to be covered in the media, well, it's not looking so good. On the one hand, there are those commendably po-faced announcements in fashion magazines that a certain $2,600 handbag is a "must have" and that the only permissible style of trousers this season is drop-crotch jodhpurs. And on the other, there are fashion commentators who make getting dressed into a kind of logic puzzle: one long torso plus two short arms equals a V-neck top with a bias-cut skirt, and if you fail to know these rules you will live your life in solitary frumpish purdah. For those of us who can barely remember how to use the coffeemaker in the morning, the thought of having to master this kind of sartorial mathematical equation before work is enough to make one want to cash in the Club Monaco gift vouchers you got for Christmas and curl up in a burlap sack.

But if you look at how women in this country actually relate to fashion, it's a very different story. Thanks largely to the rise of mass market fashion, with a special bouquet going to H&M, and also to the crop of young designers who have emerged over the past two decades, particularly Marc Jacobs; Miuccia Prada; Comme des Garcons' Rei Kawakubo; Stella McCartney, the former designer for Chloé; Phoebe Philo; Nicolas Ghesquière; and Luella Bartley, fashion is more than ever for the women themselves, not the men who look at them. It is surely no coincidence that the majority of the designers mentioned above are women.

In regard to the impact of mass market fashion, never before have so many good clothes been so readily available so cheaply, and never before have so many women been in the position to buy them with their own money. These clothes are a far cry from the itchy boob tubes, baggy jeans, and other pathetic excuses for clothes the stores shamelessly sold in the '80s. Instead, a woman can buy a fantastically smart work suit at Zara and pick up a tunic dress that makes her feel fabulous at the same time. Go into H&M on a Saturday (not something I would normally recommend—save your sanity and wait for

Sunday) and you will see gaggles of giggling teenagers and pairs of grown women, silent with concentration, diligently flicking through beautiful blouses and more-than-decent dresses, admiring themselves in the mirror and paying their own money for things that make them happy. Some might see this as a kind of nightmarish vision of materialistic hell; but unless I missed a crucial lesson in History 101, the Western world is not under Communist rule, and it is permissible for a woman to buy something, just for her, that gives her a little smile of pleasure when she sees it in the closet the next morning. The response to this view is that the only reason for that pleased smile is that, actually, the fashion press brainwashes women into thinking that they have to buy that dress, that they *need* that clutch bag, and thus any happiness is artificial, transient, and conditioned. It's an interesting contention, and one that would almost be worth responding to if it didn't take the tack that women are childlike dullards who just don't know their own minds, bless them, and need to be protected from big scary *Vogue,* which, like a villainous bounder, is stealing the life savings from doddering and gullible females across the land.

There is more to a

woman than what she wears and how she looks; of course there is. But I just do not see that having a sharp brain and strong self-esteem is incompatible with caring about how you look, and deriving pleasure from it. Surely the latter, at least, is something to be encouraged. Aside from the fact that a little dash of narcissism is human nature, the opposite contention has led to a whole generation of young women refusing to describe themselves as feminists because they equate "feminism" with excess body hair as opposed to equal rights.

The companion to the antifashion argument is, if it's not making women too happy, then it's making them too miserable. Fashion should be about making people feel good about themselves: confident, attractive, individual. But somewhere along the way it accrued a rather annoying parasitic concern—namely, body obsession. It is a real blinking shame that fashion, which exists ostensibly to give women self-confidence, has become something that many people see as precisely the opposite. Without question, the industry needs to expand its concept of the physical ideal or, even better, to lose its obsession with it. But as that doesn't seem likely to happen in the next—hmmm, let's see—decade or so, it's up to women themselves to make the choice: either you can let a few preening designers and fascistic editors ruin what is otherwise a very enjoyable pastime, or you can tell them to go jump and get back to thinking about the important things in life, such as whether a mini puffball skirt will make you look like a fabulous '80s homage or just like a lady wearing a whoopee cushion.

And anyway, I'm not entirely convinced that women feel quite as oppressed by this as the fretful media purport. Think of some of the most successful trends over the past few years: tunic dresses, ballet pumps, leggings shorts, empire-line dresses and tops, clumpy wedge shoes, boots over jeans, handbags so large and ornate they could probably be used by NASA as base camps on Mars. These are clothes that are fun to wear but are guaranteed to make no one look thinner or taller and, judging by the huge swaths of ladies who cheerfully vacuum-packed themselves into skinny jeans recently, women don't seem to mind. Whereas fashions of the past always seemed to have some kind of wearisome ulterior motive—shoulder pads in the '80s to make one look more butch in the workplace, wasp waists in the '50s to create a vision of the female form that pretty much rivals Barbie in its distance from reality—women today, with the occasional Elizabeth Hurley–esque exception, dress more than ever in a style that this book shall pithily describe as Clothes That Boys Don't Get But Girls Do. Sometimes this is to their aesthetic advantage (I refuse to believe that spinning gaily on the dance floor in a loose tunic is less attractive than a woman painfully winched into something that restricts any movement more extreme than that required to give a plaintive bleat of pain), sometimes it's not (yes, shorts and tights do make a woman look like she is mid-performance of a transgendered Hamlet—I'll grant you that one). Either way, it is a marvelous retort to yet another patronizing argument that women are unable to separate the fantasy of fashion magazines from the reality of their own lives.

Finally, despite the often baffling imperative tone that dominates fashion—Red? Good! Blue? Bad!—it is, of course, a wholly subjective pursuit. This kind of bossiness, I suspect, is part of the reason that some women still find fashion frighteningly off-putting. Sweep past the naysayers and have faith in your own taste: all that matters is whether you like it or not. For anyone out there who might still feel qualms, this book will selflessly, fearlessly demonstrate the proof of this tenet. This is by no means an exhaustive guide to the fashion world, but one built wholly on personal biases and bugbears. Nor is it filled with detailed descriptions about how one should wear which accessory and to what occasion. Sometimes, yes, those kinds of tips can be helpful. But after a while, I suspect, they simply suck away what little confidence some women already have in their own sense of style.

There are plenty of books out there that give the extensive biographical details of every single designer who ever sat behind a Singer sewing machine; instead, this guide restricts itself to talking about one designer or label for each of the fashion capitals who, for various reasons, best represents that city: Marc Jacobs for New York, Prada for Milan, and Karl Lagerfeld at Chanel for Paris. Some might disagree with those choices, some might even disagree with the choice of fashion cities, what with Mumbai, Shanghai, Berlin, and Madrid all making steps up to the plate. But then, some might also disagree with this book's beliefs that fur is wrong, wedges are right, and anyone over the age of five who wears anything from Gap Kids is deeply, deeply suspect. How passé can you get?

The
MEANING
of
SUNGLASSES

> *"Everyone who is smart says they hate fashion, that it's such a waste of time. I have asked many super-serious people, 'Then why is fashion so popular?' Nobody can answer that question."*
>
> —Miuccia Prada

> *"I probably own thirty pairs of white jeans. I'm just obsessed with them."*
>
> —Elizabeth Hurley

Accessories: going to hell in a handbag

Once upon a time, in a faraway land, the fashion world was mainly about clothes. Now, as anyone whose Brobdingnagian bag has left her with a lifetime of orthopedic bills knows, it's mainly about the accessories.

The reason more women will spend $1,400 on a Chloé handbag than they will on a Chloé dress is well known (sing it as one, sisters): a-bag-never-makes-you-feel-fat. And its appeal to designers is equally simple: it sells faster.

And it's not just about bags. Every season there seem to be more little trinkets—from Chanel camellia brooches to Miu Miu faux school crests—and one can only applaud the designers' ingenuity. Never before has fashion been quite so much about the hors d'oeuvres instead of the main meal. Once accessories operated, the way perfume still does to an extent, as a compensating taster for those who wanted a bit of designer label action yet couldn't afford to commit to a full-on relationship. But now accessories themselves have become just as expensive as the frocks because, as designers have learned, there really are some people out there who will pay $1,000 for a Marc Jacobs knitted hat.

Even at the less extreme end of the scale, why people are quite so enthralled by accessories leads one unavoidably to some ugly human truths. First, they flash the cash that little bit quicker. Swinging about a giant handbag decked with an undeniably pointless padlock will send a certain message—namely, I Can Afford Chloé—a lot faster than just wearing a pair of plain Chloé trousers. We can blame the mass market for this to an extent, because now that it has become so good at copying designer clothes, it is harder to justify buying that Marni smock when you know Zara will have a near-as-dammit one at literally one-twentieth of the price. Accessories—well, handbags and shoes, anyway—are harder to copy, particularly if, as designers have cleverly spotted, the It ones of the season are decked in chains, buckles, and silken threads strung with priceless

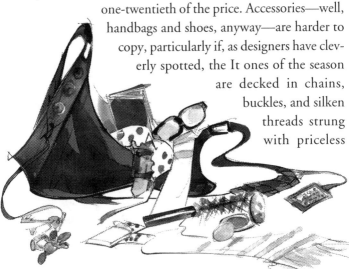

Japanese sea pearls. (An exaggeration may lurk therein, but the essential truth is unchanged.)

But as fun as it is to blame H&M for all of our capitalistic ills, the truth is that none of it would matter if there wasn't something inside many of us that wants to flaunt how much money we've spent. Thus, we'll buy all the tunic dresses we like at H&M, but, you know, a lady still wants the world to see that she can lay out the occasional $1,600, okay? If anything, the contrast between the designer accessory and mass market clothes ups your fash cred because it shows that you may have money but you spend it judiciously.

None of this is in itself necessarily a bad thing: if having that handbag or those shoes makes you happy, then why the hell not? It's your money and, as already said, if you're going to spend serious cash, it really is better to do it on the accessories because the ones on the mass market are much less well made (see **Money, and when to spend it**). And, heck, there are worse ways to show off one's wealth, such as having a customized car license plate or making small children in Colombia harvest drugs for you.

Yet there is something a tad self-deluding about this buying of accessories but shying away from the clothes. It's like believing that any food you eat while standing up and cooking doesn't count. You may as well just forgo all the little bits and save up enough for a Chanel jacket—or its calorific equivalent, the quattro formaggio—and accept that you are as much a fashion sucker as the next run-of-the-(tread)mill socialite. Yes, designer accessories may be better made than mass market ones, but let's not kid ourselves that all those extra chains and buckles and locks and contrasting threads are there for purposes even approaching practical. Moreover, the rise of the It bag proves just how much thoughts about practicality have been jettisoned. Once we justified the purchase of an expensive bag or pair of shoes by making high claims for their longevity. That phrases like "this season's must-have bag" have smoothly entered the lexicon suggests that "longevity" now means roughly six months.

The real point to notice about accessories is just how clever designers have been at reinventing the wheel—or at least suddenly adding extra spokes heretofore unnecessary to your wheel's motion. Take the "key fob" for example, which became very popular a few years ago, thanks to younger labels such as Marc by Marc Jacobs and Luella. This, to the eyes of the ignorant, is merely a key chain by another name. But, ah, they are overlooking three crucial differences: (1) It's not for your keys, but rather to clip on your oversized Mulberry bag, meaning that your $2,000 handbag now needs its own accessories. It does mean that the word "key" in the name is a little misleading but is compensated for by the unexpected accuracy of "fob," because it was, in fact, fobbed off on the public. (2) Key chains have tacky, airport souvenir stand associations that are just unacceptable to a designer. More acceptable, though, is how lucrative these little kinds of knickknacks can be. So with one single word alteration, the once unbearable has been rendered crucial. (3) They're about ten times more expensive.

The rise of accessories has intriguingly coincided with the increase of designers and decent clothing shops in general, leading one to believe that maybe, after all, we have reached a point of having enough dresses, a surfeit of trousers, just that one-too-many tops-that-go-well-with-jeans. But a Louis Vuitton feathered beret? A Marc Jacobs key fob? An Hermès muff? How have you never noticed that gaping hole in your wardrobe before? Charge it!

Advertising: how it spins the fashion axis

With perhaps the exception of the fashion assistant, who knows how the invoicing system works and where the key to the fashion cupboard is, no one has greater power in the fashion world than—any guesses? No, not the designers, bless your idealistic soul. The editors? Stop it, you're bustin' my ribs. The models' nutritionists? Score for the lateral thinking, but no. It's the boringly besuited, sweaty, balding, utterly uninterested-in-anything-to-do-with-looking-stylish advertising executives. This is not some rant against the stultifying capitalist world in which we live because no reasonable being can sustain this kind of idealistic, socialist-ish argument about an industry predicated on flogging pretty bits and bobs.

But if you have managed to hold on to your innocence and happen to have a free hour or so, try this fun experiment: go through a magazine and count how many advertisements for each brand appear; then count how many times that brand name is mentioned in the magazine, in either articles or fashion shoots; and then lean back and marvel at how they tally. In short, a magazine with an advertisement for, say, Prada on the back cover is a magazine that's going to be featuring a lot of Prada in its shoots, plus maybe an interview with Miuccia thrown in for good measure. This is known in the industry parlance as "showing support," as in, "You didn't show us enough support last season, so we're taking our annual $4 million advertising account elsewhere. Have fun picking out what to wear on the welfare line, suckers."

This is why you will never read anything negative in a fashion magazine, except, of course, something about last season, and even under those extreme circumstances, designers' names will not be mentioned. *Par exemple:* "Layers, out! Armani's frills, in!" And so, somewhat improbably, fashion magazines are actually the most cheerful publications on this planet and should probably be prescribed to depressives instead of Prozac. They are object lessons in how to see only the good in something.

It's not just the advertisers' money that keeps the mags in thrall: good advertising makes a magazine look better. A nice ad for Estee Lauder featuring Gwyneth Paltrow is going to make a magazine look more upmarket than one for Easy Spirit pumps. And as many fashion magazine articles and fashion shoots are, as everyone's mother has pointed out, indistinguishable from advertising, it's a wonder that no one has published a magazine of just advertisements, reeled in the cash from not having to pay for any journalists, editors, or photographers, and chortled all the way to an offshore tax-break private island.

But the relationship is not one-sided, and here things get a bit complex. Advertisers are as dependent on the cachet of the magazine as the magazine is on the cash of the ad. To see an advertisement for Balenciaga in, say, French *Vogue* carries a slightly different intimation or—to use the advertising lingo— "level of credibility for the brand" than if it was forced to plop itself in, say, *Us Weekly.* So despite actually funding the publication, advertisers know how much they need the scabby editors and their pesky little magazines, and God help us if they don't make editorial pay. Aside from the gushing copy, there is general obsequiousness and all sorts of other genuflections required from magazine editors: lunches with publicists and enforced attendance at even the dreariest fashion shows (see **Fashion shows: Darwin in motion**) and "press days," when the fashion writer is presented with a rack of the very same clothes she just saw in the show and, bringing back memories of school presentations for which she did not prepare, is forced to comment on them. These, along with the general puffery that makes up so much of fashion writing, are the very things that give fashion journalism a bad name, all of which are ascribable to, yes, advertising. So fine, this is a rant against advertising, albeit a suicidal one conducted in the knowledge that without advertising much of the fashion world wouldn't exist. But, hey, even suicidal socialists are allowed to be well dressed.

Animal print: when women roar

Contrary to what your mother told you, an outfit's quota of tackiness has nothing to do with the height of a hem, the inches of a heel, or the tightness of a skirt. It has to do with the obviousness of its message. Granted, the three qualities aforementioned can convey certain messages at loudspeaker level, but they are not the whole story. For example, a very tight but elongated (say, mid-calf level) pencil skirt mixes its messages and is therefore very classy in a, like, totally McQueen kinda way, whereas a super tight, super short miniskirt will have men asking if you charge by the hour. The lesson here is that you should never underestimate your audience. We have long gone past the point of just undoing that extra blouse button and entered into the generation of sloganed T-shirts. Girls, if your T-shirt has to say it, you ain't it, and if it has to say it twenty times, you never will be.

Animal-print clothing is even more grating because the message is simultaneously so embarrassingly obvious and so cringingly stupid. Yeah, we get it, babe—you're wild. In the sack, yes, yes. Like on Discovery Channel—WE GOT IT.

If the print is on actual fur, well, that is, at first glance, just about forgivable because that is how fur looks, so to complain seems churlish. But then this mood of tolerance is swiftly pushed aside upon the realization that the woman is wearing fur, and this takes the concept of unacceptable to a whole new level (see **Fur: bad**).

To see a Lycra dress dutifully printed with all those black dots in desperate emulation of a leopard's skin, in a manner vaguely akin to a raddled look-alike insisting she is the spit of her chosen ethereal icon, is to see in action the definition of the phrase "wasted effort." You can hold up as many photos of Kate Moss in her snow leopard jacket or leopard-print silk slip as you like, but you are doing nothing to argue your cause: Mossy would look good in anything; that's why she is a M-O-D-E-L (see **Models**). The rest of us, however, look like craggy ol' lushes propping up the bar in a local dive, occasionally goosing the local boys and telling the snickering youths how all the men in town were once after our virtue.

Ankle boots: so wrong and yet, and yet

Here is what boots are supposed to do: keep you warm, look smart, provide ease of mobility, and be comfortable. Here is what ankle boots do: absolutely none of the above.

There is no denying that, as footwear goes, ankle boots are pretty much up there with high-heeled sneakers in terms of silliness. They make you look like a member of the cloven hoof species, they are surprisingly hard to walk in owing to lack of—despite the name—ankle support, and they go with only about two pieces of clothing, namely, knee-length or above dresses, particularly tunics, and the occasional short skirt, both of which have to be worn with tights, unless you are going for the reality-TV, girl-band look this season. Trousers with ankle boots will prompt wits to ask if little piggy is going to market, particularly if the trousers are cropped or, sweet Jesus, tucked into the boots. And yet, unlike high-heeled sneakers, ankle boots make one come over all Fatboy Slim in wanting to praise them, like we do.

Yes, they look ridiculous. And, yes, your calves will resemble stuffed sausages. However, sometimes a woman just doesn't—gasp!—care if something makes her look like Scarlett Johansson or not (see **Get: fashion that girls do and boys don't**). For a start, ankle boots are a glorious alternative to their more mainstream mother ship, knee-length boots, which are always useful but occasionally dull, not to mention sweaty (see **Boots: the normal kind with a couple of variations**). Ankle boots, however, suggest that the wearer is no safe, mainstream, probably-a-fan-of-Coldplay kinda lady. Oh no, forget about Gwyneth Paltrow, we got Courtney Love over here, gentlemen. And fine, perhaps Courtney is not everywoman's life counselor but, damn, it would be pretty boring to eat mung beans every day. And most important of all, they're fun to dance in. This makes them pretty much unique in the world of female footwear. They may not provide as much support as normal boots but are more stable than heels and just more of a laugh than flats. Thus, they are one of the few benefits of the near annual '80s fashion revivals, just about compensating for the accompanying jumper dresses (scratchy and surprisingly unflattering) and designer hair scrunchies (elaboration unnecessary) that emerge with them.

Antiaging

In this super snazzy, techno-happy, come-and-watch-a-brain-transplant-on-my-HDTV-while-I-download-some-bootleg-Japanese-films-on-my-iPhone age of ours, we like to think we've come a long way from the superstitious, leech-happy Middle Ages. The fact that the skin-care industry rakes in billions of dollars a year proves we have definitely not. Frankly, it's a miracle we no longer tie women over forty to a stake in the town square and burn them. (We're much more sensible: we just ignore the old crones.) In centuries gone by doctors informed their trusting patients that removing their blood from their weakened bodies would cure them; in the twenty-first century we believe a C-list celebrity when she tells us that a pot of white cream made partly from whale sperm but mainly from a load of chemicals will literally "reverse time." That's progress, baby!

Skin care suggests many perfectly commendable things: curing acne, resolving rosacea, simply giving your face a good scrub. But none of these seem quite exciting enough to explain the monolithic skin-care industry. Skin care is so huge that it is often the supporting scaffolding of a fashion house, sopping up debts incurred by an unprofitable clothes division, it being much easier to convince the plebs to shell out $60 for a tub of gunk than $1,400 for a tweed jacket. Yet the tweed jacket gives the brand name the allure that sells the gunk, even though you didn't really want the jacket in the first place. Don't think about this too long or the entire fashion skeleton will develop osteoporosis and crumble.

There are only three things in this world that make people spend collective billions: the promise of power, of sex, or of looking thinner or younger. Obviously, you will get the first two only if you are the latter, so guess which one people seem to care most about these days. "Skin care" is now a euphemism for making oneself look younger, just as "detox" is a fancy word for dieting with an extra $20 for a bunch of organic carrots instead of a $2 calorie counter (see **Yoga, detoxes, and other euphemisms for exercise and diets**).

Why we all care so much about looking young is a bit of a puzzle. In the Middle Ages this veneration of the young was understandable, mainly because if you reached thirty you were pretty much knocking on heaven's door, so sixteen, to use the inverse neologism beloved by many a women's magazine, was the new fifty, and women had to get themselves knocked up ASAP to continue the human race. But now that a woman can have a child at fifty-eight and we're told there are too many of us around anyway, the increasing hysteria about the value of youth does seem odd. The press continues to make happy hay on a slow news day by printing a photo of someone in the public eye from twenty years ago next to one of them today, showing that they—no, it cannot be!—look twenty years older. Time has passed! Stop the presses!

Maybe it has to do with that irksomely childish, if endearingly reliable, human trait of always wanting something that you cannot have. Or maybe we are all living in the movie *Logan's Run*, and no one noticed because we're missing the white suits and Michael York. Or maybe it's because we're foolish enough to have been brainwashed by a moneygrubbing beauty industry eagerly grasping at our waving dollars. Who can say?

Happily, the skin-care industry has stepped up to this much-needed plate, flogging tubs of godknowswhat to the desperate public, like a medicine man proffering worm claw and cats' nipples to a country town riddled with plague. In 2005, America alone spent over $660 million on antiaging products. Now ask yourself if Americans are looking any younger these days.

Plastic surgery and Botox are a separate issue in that there is no faffing about with pretty euphemisms here, no pretending you're just "looking after your skin." No, we're talking "Get the scalpel and needle out, doctor, and slice up my face" level of bluntness here (see **Plastic surgery, and how all those 1950s B movies weren't so far off the mark**). Botox is rather like hard drugs in that it may have the immediately desired effect, but this is only short-lived, and you'll find yourself on a treadmill of injections, having to top yourself up with annoying frequency. The fact that you can't make any facial expression is another deterrent, though perhaps that's how the people who advocate the treatment maintain a straight face.

The very word "antiaging" gives the game away, that this must be the most fruitless cause since Ross Perot for president. It brings to mind, funnily enough, the chosen slogan of the anti-abortion lobby ProLife, although, as the genius that was Bill Hicks once said, if they were all so pro-life, instead of picketing hospitals maybe they should protest against cemeteries. A similar point could be made about this antiaging malarkey, as the only thing that will stop anyone from looking a day older than they did yesterday is—insert drumroll—death. Yet rather than sign the Grim Reaper, cosmetics companies seem to prefer currently resting representatives from the acting community. Although considering that moisturizers are made from a load of alphabet-heavy chemicals, most of which will probably turn out to be highly carcinogenic, maybe they are onto something here.

Bags: a word or ten thereon

That women love bags is a fact for which the fashion business gives a collective hallelujah to the god of capitalism on a daily basis (see **Accessories: going to hell in a handbag**). Why they love bags is for pretty much the same reasons they love shoes: they don't make you feel fat, you don't have to get undressed to try them on, size is either a nonissue or simply not related to your stomach, and they don't necessarily suit Kate Moss any better than you, all of which is basically saying the same thing four different ways. Women try to justify this love affair with high claims about "being able to use a bag more than you would use one dress." This claim loses some currency as you buy your sixth handbag. Furthermore, surely this is more true about, say, a coat, but coats have yet to send women into apoplexies of pleasure in the way that bags do (see **Coats: stuck at the nexus between dull and stressful**).

So if the bag has become a statement, then one is duty-bound to decode the buyer's individual meanings. After all, if a woman spends $1,200 on a leather good, the least one can do is try to figure out what she is attempting to say, other than, of course, "I've spent over a grand on something in which to keep my dirty Kleenex and a defluffed lip-gloss brush."

Because you have to hold a structured handbag in, as the name does suggest, your hand, this is an accessory that screams, "I never have to carry my own shopping! Valet service all the way, babycakes!" Thus, to the majority of the human race, it is of no use whatsoever (see **Clutch "bag"**). You want to carry home more than one load of groceries? Outrageous! Not with the bag that will put 50 percent of your available hands out of commission. You will spend your life trying to shove that mean little strap up your lower arm in an attempt to liberate your hand, but your victory can only be short-lived. Thus are you forced to surrender to the tyranny of the handbag.

Satchel bags are very useful for pretending that you are Ali MacGraw, circa 1976. But despite that indisputable advantage, they are one of the many garments on this planet not made for anyone with the temerity to grow herself a pair of breasts. (Hippie chicks didn't have breasts. They were too busy making daisy chains to grow them. This is why there is not a single item of clothing from the late '60s to early '70s that accommodates them. The good reader is referred to the contemporary works of Yves Saint Laurent and Ossie Clarke, not to mention the veneration of the young Mia Farrow, should she require further proof.) Thus, like the blouse (see **Blouses: not so librarian**

now, are they?), they work best for those who use theirs to carry home French homework, rather than those toting BlackBerrys and office work and broken Tampax. You can just let the satchel dangle down as opposed to crossing it over your chest, traffic-warden-style, but it will bang against your thigh something chronic, and you may as well just hand your wallet to a passing pickpocket and have done with it.

So make like Goldilocks and get one with a strap that is not too short, not too long, but just right, i.e., one that can be shoved up onto your shoulder or gripped in your hand as the whim takes you. Don't be an idiot and get one in suede or cotton or canvas or whatever kind of nonwaterproof fabric. A bag you have to worry about getting dirty is as stupid as shoes you cannot walk in and screams only one thing: sucker.

Which designer made your bag says even more about you than does its style—veritable proof that we have long since left the land of practicalities and entered a world of statements. Because designers and customers can have more fun with bags than clothes—free from having to worry about inconvenient things like women's bodies—the bag, more than any other piece of fashion, is used to solidify a brand's image and what customers use to be part of it. Bags communicate these signals faster than clothes because, simply, they are more ostentatious.

Chloé's Edith bag might look at first like the kind of thing Miss Gulch might have shoved in her bicycle basket in *The Wizard of Oz*, but its message is the same as that of the brand's younger-looking Paddington: namely, that the customer is (or fancies herself to be) a young and sassy lady, who probably lives in some very cool loft in the city with her very cool boyfriend but just loves to go riding at Mummy's on the weekends. Maybe she bought that battered leather bag from a vintage store, maybe it was a legacy from her quasi-aristocratic grandmother. More likely, she coughed up more that $1,000 on Fifth Avenue.

Fendi, on the other hand, with its sharp and shiny logos, is about frighteningly well groomed and even more frighteningly well monied Continental ladies who use words like "chinchilla" and "arctic fox" on a daily basis. Thanks to the genius of Karl Lagerfeld, Chanel bags now send multiple signals: either I am a trashy starlet being ironic or I am a lady who lunches at Le Caprice and I still think it's 1986 or I know my fashion history and I only accept the best (aka, the most expensive). Contrary to industry belief that multiple signals dilute appeal, Lagerfeld actually just tripled his potential customers, and that's why he is the kaiser (see **Lagerfeld, Karl, and why he's so brilliant**). These brand images are created partly by the bags themselves but also by a combination of advertising, magazine puffery, and "product placement," better known as which celebrities are chosen to be given the bag for free.

Superfluous hardware on the bag has become another favored form of branding in recent years and has proven enormously popular with customers, despite making the bag weigh about the same as a small car, and that's before you've put anything in it. The attraction lies mainly in that all these excess buckles, chains, and padlocks shout the bag's label name without any logo names, which are far too obvious and therefore vulgar, whereas a whopping great lock and key, which serves absolutely no purpose other than to prove that the bag is Chloé, is the height of good taste. And really, a lifetime of osteopaths' bills is surely a small price to pay for chic.

There have been some rather interesting theories around about how the rise of accessory hardware coincides with international unrest and, um, a general sense of insecurity and, um, yeah. Personally, I love this theory. So all those Marc Jacobs chains, Mulberry buckles, and Anya Hindmarch rivets aren't indicative of being fashion victims? No, we're doing our bit for our country, to free those hearts and minds! Yeah! Yet one cannot help but wonder whether this attempt to claim that our materialism benefits international aid and Dubya's great cause might put women off the bags in a way that the price tags don't seem to do.

You can find perfectly decent bags on the mass market, but they tend to look like they're made either for thirteen-year-olds or for one-hundred-and-three-year-olds, yet another reason more women are forking out for designer handbags. Plus, you probably will give your bag more of a battering than you will, for example, a summer dress, so perhaps it is worth spending a little bit more on something that is well made and won't fall apart after three outings and one rainfall. So yes, there is a smidgen of a practical justification here. But only a smidgen, mind.

As for men, despite designers' and men's magazines' best attempts, the man bag has never really caught on, not only because of the name's almost offensive stupidity but also because the majority have to be carried (see, again, **Clutch "bag"**). Rucksacks are permissible only if you are at a music festival, under twenty-five, or Australian—ideally, all three. Briefcases are fine, if not exactly the wildest option in town, and as for a computer bag, well, that is just sooooo late '90s. So embrace your lack of mammaries and get a handy little satchel bag, which

for some unfair reason won't endow you with the hippie connotations. Not that there's anything wrong with hippies, 'course,
peace, love, and all that. But we're talking about bags here, okay?
And some things just obviously take precedence.

Ballet pumps: twee versus comfort

The trajectory of a trend from Moss to mass to verboten is both
swift and cruel. To recap, Kate Moss wears something, she gets
photographed, the world trembles with excitement, the mass
market rolls up its plagiarizing sleeves, and—bada bing, bada
boom—what was once so maverick now reeks of D-list celebrity
photo ops and sullen teens in H&M (see **Moss, Kate, and how
she ruined your wardrobe**).

Ballet pumps were always destined to be the archetypal
victims of this sad descent because of the Gorgon-like curse of
(a) looking very good on Kate Moss, (b) being extraordinarily
easy for the mass market to copy, but (c) trickier than you'd
think to do well.

When Moss was first photographed wearing them a few years
ago, ah, how she brought back the memories, which we shall
recap here in not particularly zeitgeisty Quentin Tarantino fast-
editing form: Hepburn! Bardot! Gamine! Skinny cropped trousers! Bang! Gore! Pointless diversion into '70s cultural in-joke!
Anyone who hasn't been blinded by the ingenuity of this technique will have noticed that the common denominator of all the
above is slimness, and, as ballet pumps—a footwear invented
for, lest we forget, the not-exactly-girthsome demographic of
ballet dancers—show, just because something emphasizes a thin
person's svelteness does not mean it will make you look thin.

This is a truth that the success of skinny jeans proves has yet to be understood. Of course, this doesn't actually matter; after all, if we looked like Kate Moss, then we wouldn't be quite so thrilled by photos of her appearing a bit spotty with whatever droopy boyfriend she's currently squiring, and what a poorer world this would be. And to be honest, a curvy woman trotting about with a smile in a pair of simple flats is a far more attractive sight than a twiglet limping miserably in stilettos, but we'll get back to that in a bit.

It's not rounded calves that have been ballet pumps' downfall but their cheap imitators. Despite their apparent simplicity, ballet pumps are very easy to get wrong. In fact, the simpler the concept, the easier it is to do badly, as pretty much every spin-off TV show has proven, with the notable exception of *Frasier*.

The perfect ballet pumps have delicately rounded toes: not squat and wide ones like the cap of a mushroom but ones with a gently rounded point. The soles should be thin and can be either soft or—for a more formal (and longer-lasting) look— hard, which is a style that the company French Sole has made its own. They need to be narrow, as otherwise you will look like a little duck padding down toward the pond, and they should cut away just past the division of your toes. Always go for solid colors, though be wary of red, as people will just keep asking you if there's no place like home. And be careful about metallics, because if you wear gold ballet pumps with black tights someone might mistake you for a grand piano, which would just be awkward for everyone.

In other words, ballet pumps should look as much like— ooh, what a shocker—proper ballet slippers as possible, albeit not in pink (see **Pink**). The originals really are the best; that's why we ripped them off in the first place (see **Classics with a twist**).

Squared toes, thick soles, rain-damaged tips, gratingly girly colors, and patterns of the hot pink polka-dot, little animal, and shooting-star variety have decimated ballet pumps' once proud, understated, Left Bank–chic image. Truly, shoes with cartoon kittens on them have never crossed the threshold of Café de Flore. Instead, ballet pumps have become the prissy, water-logged alternative to sneakers.

All that said, the ultimate reason the world took to ballet pumps is because they are really, really, really comfortable, a sensation women experience all too rarely south of their ankles. With the exception of sneakers and the occasional flat boot, they are the closest women have come to finding an acceptable shoe that gives them an insight into what it feels like to be a man, able to walk with nary a limp nor risk of bloodletting. Admittedly, they do suffer from weather-dependent issues, but still, as (possible) ballet pump connoisseur Meat Loaf once so wisely said, two out of three ain't bad. And the word of Mr. Loaf, as he really is known to his many respectful followers, unquestionably trumps any aesthetic quibbles. Except the cartoon kittens, of course.

Bathing suits, and how so little can reveal so much

There is a general belief, propagated primarily by daytime TV shows and women's magazines, that the reason beach holidays are, to use their favored term, so "stressful" is the body exposure they require. Certainly, the first day on the beach can be a little "stressful" if you have any neuroses about your body, pasty skin, or surplus body hair. But pretty much by lunchtime you realize that, actually, the beach is a fantastic leveler. Forget about religious pilgrimages or dawn epiphanies: there ain't nothing like a day on the beach to restore your faith in an omniscient and wise Creator. Almost no one has a perfect body, and no one really cares. There they all sit in the beach café, tummies hanging over their waistbands, happily asking for extra ketchup with their fries. For heaven's sake, you spent all this money on a holiday, are you really going to waste it by mentally angsting over something magazines insist on calling "love handles," aka skin? But conversely, those who do have perfect bodies and have yet to experience the novel sensation of their bottom rubbing against their mid-thighs are almost invariably so unappealing in some way that one cannot help but pity them, not envy them. If they are male, they will almost always be utterly stupid, dull, or vain, those being the necessary qualities of a man who bothered to cultivate the body beautiful, who will spend the day obtrusively walking up and down the beach in the apparent belief that this is a very subtle way to garner admiration. (This is one of the disadvantages of being stupid: you always underestimate your audience.) If you are a woman, either you will be so heavily composed of plastic that you'll have to hide indoors to keep from melting in the midday sun, or you will be on the arm of a cigar-chomping hairy beast, who definitely does not have a perfect body, and people will secretly refer to you as "the geisha" behind your back; or you will be very stupid and will annoy everyone on the beach by talking loudly on your cell about your latest colonic and going to Sundance with "Leo." Or possibly all three. Yes, God is good.

It's one thing when you have clothes on, because then you can do some judicious covering, should you be so inclined. On the beach, you just gotta let it all hang out and be Zen. The fact that many women choose to wear bikinis instead of one-pieces pretty much proves that, at least on the beach, women might not be quite as neurotic about their bodies as is generally assumed and perhaps all the fuss about having a flat stomach isn't quite as important as one has always been led to believe.

Choosing what to wear on the beach, however, is a trickier matter because here you do have control. Designer swimwear is obviously for people who have no intention of swimming (see **Exercise clothes: the new couture**), and that makes sense. If they're going to be on full display all day above sea level, they might as well spend money on making sure that everyone can see they're sporting the new Missoni colors this season on their bikini. Bathing suits with comedy cutouts are just funny. Aside from the obvious tan line issues, it's one thing to have some cheeky cutouts on a long, demure evening dress, but when a woman's in a bathing suit and the rest of her body is pretty much on display anyway, somehow getting a triangular view of her lower ribs, say, doesn't quite have quite the same impact.

A woman in a one-piece bathing suit is either a professional swimmer, someone with issues about the shape of her tummy, or someone traumatized by a missing bikini top incident. If you reside in any of these catergories, fine; just make sure you get a swimsuit with defined cups at the top, as one-piece bathing suits bind you like Yentl. String bikinis are for the very confident and the very flat-chested (i.e., plastic trophy girlfriends and models on holiday); for everyone else, a bit of support is always welcome, as the Samaritans might very well say. Unusually, the fashion compromise for bathing suits actually works quite well: the tankini—basically, a waterproof camisole top with matching bottoms—and gets the best of both, in that there is a bit of stomach coverage without the breast bind, and therefore it says the wearer might have a few body issues, but she is not going to let this ruin her holiday.

Occasionally you'll see a bikini with a slightly frilled skirt attached to the bottom that's meant to hide "a multitude of sins"—having chomped through three Polly-O String Cheeses last week obviously being on a par with murder, adultery, and coveting your neighbor's (nondimpled) ass. However, the obviously infantalizing nature of this garment, making it fall well under the umbrella of pedophile chic (see **Mittens, and the enduring appeal of pedophile-friendly chic**), pretty much cancels out any other benefits. Fifties-style swimsuits, in which the bottoms are cut higher on the tummy and lower under the bum, are often recommended for similar reasons and, again, there is logic here. That these swimsuits allow you to let your bikini line go for a little bit longer is another benefit, albeit one rarely mentioned by *Vogue*. They will, however, make one resemble a wartime pinup, and you may feel like you should be straddling a nuclear bomb and painted on the side of a plane.

Black is obviously the most flattering color for swimwear, hence the reason it is the only color you ever see Kate Moss sporting, making one wonder for a few schadenfreude-freighted moments if maybe she isn't that hot after all, considering she clings so neurotically to slimming back. However, while Kate might not see a beach holiday as that big a deal, seeing as she seems to be on at least one every month, most of the rest of the human species probably wouldn't mind marking the occasion with a color a little more celebratory than such a funereal shade.

Solid colors are generally recommended simply because you won't tire of them as quickly during your bathing suit's lifetime (average life span: six summer holidays—nine, if you can really stretch the elastic out).

Because the canvas is much smaller, so to speak, any messages thereon come across that much stronger and louder. Thus, a leopard-print bikini is doubly unacceptable unless you are starring in *The Return of the 50-Foot Woman* (see **Animal print: when women roar**). One-piece bathing suits with wavy lines around the waist area meant to give an illusion of slimness are about as subtle as Tom Cruise's grin, and any superfluous details—dangling chains, tassels, belts—are the equivalent of surplus baggage for a weekend away: unnecessary extras that will weigh down what should be a simple, hands-free affair. Have fun on the beach, by all means, but maybe it's best to avoid pink Pucci bikinis with full-length tassels, restricting that fun to the piña coladas and wave jumping.

Beauty treatments, and the etiquette thereof

It is usually around the time when you are lying naked as the day you first greeted the world atop a towel-covered surgeon's table, sounds of the ocean playing maddeningly on loop, your skin covered in some kind of viscous goop, a stranger's hands slipping perilously ever further down your back while she asks you merrily, "Ooh, what's this funny bruise here?" that one thinks, Now, how would Emily Post behave in this situation?

Beauty treatments are not a wholly modern phenomenon—ladies have been advised to take the waters since Roman times—but their huge variety and lack of medical purpose is. Once massages were what boxers received from their tobacco-chewing managers in between bouts; now they are something women bleat about needing at the end of a long day of work, dreaming about a darkened room, Eastern fusion music, and the strong hands of a woman called Hilda.

And all this is to the good. Women love expensive beauty treatments even if, as most suspect, they don't really yield any long-term results. As with reading fashion magazines, sometimes it's just nice to take an hour and do something that's just about oneself (see, **Magazines, fashion, and women's masochistic love thereof**). But massages have thrown up quite a slew of questions about decorum. How does one know if one is to get fully undressed or just take off one's coat? And if you are to get fully undressed, does that mean fully undressed? Should you try to befriend the person who is now intimate with your innermost crevices? Oh Emily, how the women of Madison Avenue long for your guidance.

First, be nice to your therapist. This might seem obvious, but your natural shyness on meeting them might be mistaken for coldness. So look them in the eye, smile, greet them by name, and at least pretend you're listening to them when they start blathering on about the youth-giving properties of yucca-tree oil. The nicer you are, the less likely it is they'll giggle with their colleagues later about the funny pimple on the inside of your upper thigh. Don't make any self-deprecating jokes about why you're getting this treatment. For one, if you start putting yourself down, the therapist will feel free to make similarly harsh comments about the state of your body mid-treatment, a subject we'll return to with vehemence later. And for another, it will probably sound like you're making fun of the beauty industry as a whole, and mocking someone's career is generally not a good start to a relationship.

How much you should take off depends on you and the treatment. Full-body massage—let it all hang out; for an eye treatment, you can leave your hat (and everything else) on. But whatever you're going for, don't be bullied into taking off more than you want to. It's your treatment, after all. Do accept that the more you leave on, the more garments you'll have to get dry-cleaned once they're covered with oil. Many people hesitate to get naked out of bodily shame. Although one is loath to draw the comparison between the transaction one has with a beauty therapist and that between prostitute and client, it is inescapably apt. Not only has the beauty therapist seen far worse bodies than yours but also they're not really looking at your body anyway— they see it as simply that of another client from whom they are getting their next $120. So stop being so self-obsessed; nobody cares but you. Feel free to tell them if their wretched "Sounds of the Jungle" compilation is getting on your nerves. Just say you prefer silence so you can concentrate on the treatment. Quite why almost all beauty treatment places insist on having this Indothaijapanesechinajungle mélange has never been fully explained. Maybe it's because there are few things that will make you more in need of another massage than being forced to listen to toucans for ninety minutes and then enduring the embarrass-ment of seeing your masseuse—typically, a twenty-year-old aspiring American Idol from Detroit—bang some bronze cym-bal over your half-naked body.

Possibly it's because the suggestion of exoticism will silence any doubts regarding the efficacy of the most dubious-sounding treat-ments—it's, like, ethnic, right?—and will imbue the client with faith in the noble wisdom of the Long Island therapist. It is a similar pose adopted by the only other sort of beauty treatment centers: the ascetically medical, in which every surface is metallic and the therapists walk around in white robes, as if you were about to have a lobotomy as opposed to a citrus-oil hand and foot massage.

No matter how fearsomely superior the ambience, don't be bullied into silence if there's something about the treatment itself you don't like. Just say if that "warming" oil is actually scalding or the "soothing" massage is causing you internal organ bruising.

Whether or not you wish to strike up a conversation and develop some kind of personal relationship is up to you. Personally, I opt for polite but silent anonymity, as I find it slightly embarrassing hearing about someone's child-care problems as they studiously give me a bikini wax, but then that might just be my prudish nature. Others believe that familiarity breeds better treatments, but I am a little skeptical about the idea that telling someone about your problems at work will encourage them to give you a better massage. More likely, they'll just give you a faster one to get you the hell off their table. The truth is, most therapists would far prefer a tip than a chat and so, as is often the way of the world, a sly twenty is probably the swifter route to a beautiful relationship.

Most people shell out for a beauty treatment in the belief it will make them feel better about themselves, the sweet naïve fools. Accept now that you will probably leave feeling a heck of a lot worse. Oh sure, you will be moisturized, oiled, dehaired, and cleansed, but you will have encountered the cruel sadism that is known as The Beauty Therapist's Banter. The beauty therapist is a species of mankind more cruel than a gynecologist's assistant ("I promise this won't hurt. You may, though, feel some discomfort . . ."), and we all have our own horror story. One friend settled herself down to a harmless massage only to hear the giggling observation, "Oh! Very pimply!" Another went for a facial, and as the facialist peered closely at her skin she asked my friend, "So, how old are you? Forty-three? Forty-five?" overestimating by almost a decade. My own is that I went for a facial and was promptly informed that my face was sagging downward—mirror held up with accompanying fingers indicating the trajectory of movement—and, my God, the state of my dark circles meant that unless I had some laser surgery RIGHT NOW I would resemble W. H. Auden at the end of his life before the year was out. At the time, I was under a quarter of a century. Almost all therapists do this, whether it's telling you that your back muscles are "a mess" or your blackheads "terrible." Some might see it as the tax one pays for vanity, but I'd have thought that the price one forks out for these treatments was sufficient recompense. Instead, obviously, they do this to get you to sign up for more treatments. (Unsurprisingly, the laser treatment I was recommended just happened to be offered by the therapist who was so urgently recommending it—a bargain at $1,200 per session, ten sessions recommended.) In the cold, non-wind-chimed light of normal day you know this. But when you are at your most vulnerable, lying naked and prone on a stranger's table as they pore over your face with a seemingly practiced eye, it's hard not to take their pronouncements as disinterested gospel. Don't get hysterical, allow these words to burn themselves into your heart, and sign up for all the recommended treatments. Thank them politely, get dressed, and leave. The whole point of beauty treatments is to have an hour or so of self-indulgence. If they start to become some form of self-punishment, with you constantly chasing the next one to head off more (real or imagined) signs of age, you have lost sight of the original point and one day will read about the latest A-list celebrity who takes her facialist with her on holiday and, instead of hooting with derision, will feel resentful that you don't have the money to do the same.

For this reason, I find that earplugs are the one essential I must bring to a beauty treatment. Thus, not only will you not hear the latest deathly warnings about the condition of your body but also you won't have to listen to the opening spiel about the efficacy of the products you are about to be lucky enough to experience (at $120 an hour). And, of course, they're just marvelous for blocking out the wind chimes.

Best-dressed lists: the myths and the madness

Fashion magazines are, it hardly needs stating, compiled according to the most rigorous of scientific and mathematical formulae, with every theory and statement repeatedly tested by independent adjudicators to ensure that everything printed, from what the new trouser length is that month to whether Sienna's new haircut is good or not, is sure to be the God's only truth.

But the annual best-dressed lists, those cheap page fillers of which magazines are ever so fond, do have, it is probably fair to say, a touch of the subjective to them. At least countdowns in other fields—music, for example—tend to have some kind of backing figures behind them. Even the magazine editors would agree: after all, they cry, they're only stating their opinion. But it's what this opinion is regarding that is the sticking point. As any reader knows who has ever been baffled by some of the stuffy old socialites who get lauded in these lists or has puzzled over the reason why when one starlet wears a certain dress it's good but when another wears the same frock it's bad, this editorial opinion has much less to do with the clothes than it does with the people wearing them.

The main boon of the best-dressed list for a magazine is that it is a remarkably easy way to suck up to someone whom the editor would like to interview one day (hence the enduring popularity of Jemima Khan and any young woman dating a member of the royal family), to justify to readers in advance next month's cover star (the reliable presence of the latest Bond girl or yet another Rolling Stone offspring), or just to feature people who make pretty pictures (any model). It is also a very good way to slag off anyone who has had the gumption to turn down an interview from the magazine or who shares an agent with someone else who has done just that. So far, not much to do with the clothes.

But then, being well dressed today doesn't have much to do with the clothes anyway. Most celebrities who get lauded with the title can't seem to get dressed period, let alone dressed well, seeing as they have a stylist on their daily payroll. Not so much best dressed, then, as best picker of a decent stylist, which, admittedly, doesn't make quite as snappy a cover line. The fact that Kate Moss does manage to figure out for herself which Bella Freud jumper should go with which Superfine jeans on a daily basis is often reported in tones of awe one might expect for the news that the model is able to decode the Rosetta stone.

But no matter, because if magazines love these kinds of countdowns, the general public loves them even more. America loves countdowns in general. This is, lest we forget, the country with entire TV stations dedicated to such matters 24/7, from "Hollywood's 100 Hottest Couples!" to, and often not deviating all that much in the lineup, "Hollywood's 100 Nastiest Divorces!"

It's not that anyone really cares, or even remembers, whom *Snobby Snob* or *Wow!* magazines decree to be the best-dressed chicken in the coop; it's just further proof that an increasingly large part of fashion's appeal to the public is seeing it worn by good-looking people with recognizable faces. The use of the countdown gives this national obsession a kind of competitive, even Roman, justification. It is as though we are not just looking at twelve pages of exciting people like Tory Burch and Lisa Rinna walking various red carpets to parties celebrating the launch of a new mobile phone handset, but rather the conclusive word on a yearlong debate, even if that debate is whose stylist wangled the best clothes out of the most fashion press offices.

Black: the new and the old

In one of the many instances in which the fashion world is like the Masons (the rituals, the odd personalities, the vague feelings of disdain toward the general public), the members within have certain tests they use to ascertain who is In and who is Out. Heel heights, trouser cuts, and other telltale fashion signs are, of course, all quickly perused upon the initial encounter but are not fail-safe indicators simply because quite a few fashion people, the most die-hard, in fact, take a kind of ironic pride in not following every trend to the letter (see **Signature style**). Instead, the surest way for someone to show that they are outside the sacred circle is to abuse the industry's mother tongue (see **Fashionspeak**), and the biggest abuse of all is to talk about The New Black. Non-fashion people love this phrase because it combines a useful hyperbole with a pleasing bit of nonsense while simultaneously mocking the fashion world's reputation for factually impossible non sequiturs. Thus, it is most commonly used in news stories discussing the popularity of something unexpected, as in, "Cycling is the new black" and "Is Barack Obama the new black?" The words "cake," "having," and "eating" come to mind a bit here.

This cliché may have once been coined by someone in the fashion world, but it is now almost never used by anyone in it. Partly because they have been shamed out of doing so, but largely because they know there will never be another black. Ah, blessed shade that makes you slimmer, goes with everything, and is also just a little bit scary—glory, glory be! Oh, fools who think any color could ever stand in its stead!

Certainly the fashion industry is always looking for another way to get people to spend their money, but even they know that claiming magenta is the new black will not convince anyone to dash off and buy a pair of $300 magenta trousers from Joseph. Instead, they'll just tell you it's "the color of the season," thereby at least acknowledging that you will only be fooled into wearing them for six months at most before those catcalls of "Yo, Bozo! The circus left town yesterday!" from the kids across the street begin to sink in.

And anyway, does anyone want a new black? For all of its above-listed benefits, some of us feel that there is too much black around as it is, with far too many women dressing themselves in shadows for our postfeminist liking. As a wise sage once said, if everybody looked the same, we'd get tired of looking at each other, and some of us definitely do. So sod the black, and sod whatever the new one is, and get out there and wear your magenta trousers with pride! Um, yeah!

Blahnik, Manolo

Like Tampax, the word "Manolo" has practically become a generic term in itself, although he perhaps would not be overly thrilled by the comparison. Venerated by the fashion cognoscenti, immortalized by *Sex and the City*, Manolo Blahnik's shoes are a rather strange proposition, being either innocuously plain (if you're looking for a pair of all but invisible strappy sandals, why then, my dear woman,

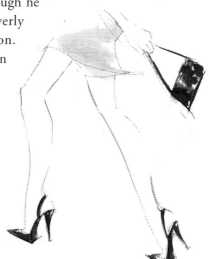

look no further, and have your $900 at the ready) or insanely over the top. This is because Blahnik has determinedly retained total independence, unlike many of his contemporaries, who have taken the conglomerate shekel and been bought up by the big fashion cartels like LVMH and the Gucci Group, and therefore can do as he darn well pleases. But the reason the term "Manolos" has become part of the lingo is that his shoes are so improbably, if admittedly only relatively, comfortable. It's about the placement of the (generally very high) heel and the angle of the instep, which should follow that of your foot. This will hold your foot in place instead of letting it slip to the bottom, jamming your toes at the tip and forcing all the weight onto the ball of your foot. The heel, meanwhile, should be placed at such an angle to allow you to put some of your weight back onto it. Otherwise, one ends up with what is known in the business as the stiletto strut, when the woman's hips are back in a different zip code from her legs because all of her weight is forced forward and she is trying in vain—"vain" being the operative word here—to find her center of balance. Moreover, Manolos last for absolute ages, which, yes, you would hope for from a shoe with an $800-plus price tag but is most certainly not something you can take for granted from designer shoes. Thus, the success of Manolo Blahnik provides us with a surprising insight into perhaps the truth of much of the fashion industry and the people who work in it: they may look all scary with their high and mighty pointy shoes, but actually they are as prone to aching arches and heel breakages as—to use Elizabeth Hurley's endlessly fascinating term for people who aren't her, Elton, or Hugh—"civilians" are, and get just as annoyed when the heel splits. And the fact that Mr. Blahnik is single-handedly keeping alive the ducktail coiffure is yet another reason to stand and applaud.

Blouses: not so librarian now, are they?

Not, of course, that there's anything wrong with librarians. But with the memorable exception of Marian, the librarian in *The Music Man,* this is not a profession that has garnered particularly seductive associations. Nor, until recently, has the blouse. This poor garment was a victim of, first, film stereotyping when it became wardrobe shorthand for mousy little repressed secretary ("buttoned up," you see—clever!), followed by trends prejudice: it was too old-fashioned for the youthful '60s, too starchy for the floppy '70s, too delicate for the shoulder-padded and tailored '80s, and too fussy for the grungy '90s. But the noughties, as we are reluctantly forced to call the decade of 2000–2009, has yet to decide on its adjectival epitaph, so the blouse has managed to slip back on in there.

Chloé can take a lot of the credit for this because this brand showed that, actually, the blouse is as flirtatious as a fantasy convent girl. Unlike a boring old T-shirt, the blouse lets you play with its near-but-still-modest transparency, by wearing either a camisole or a respectable bra beneath it, ideally without deodorant stains; you can adjust the cleavage factor, thanks to the buttons, meaning it is perhaps one of only four garments on this planet that really can be worn, to use that much trumpeted phrase, day to night (the others being, as most women have figured out, a wrap dress, good jeans, and decent boots); it looks a lot smarter than your average top, and it often looks better untucked, meaning you get tummy coverage without the slob factor.

Yes, well, hurrah, hurrah, thank heavens for the resurrection of the blouse, la-di-da, what took us so long, et cetera, and so on. Well, painful as it is to admit, our ancestors in the '80s and beyond weren't wholly unevolved in their thinking. The blouse ain't brilliant.

Don't get one in a sepia hue or with some kind of old-fashioned haberdashery pattern on it: you think you're making an ironic fashion statement; in fact you just look like Miss Marple. (And while we're here, a word about "ironic" fashion statements: irony is a tone that is best delivered orally, not visually. Thus the majority of "ironic" fashion statements tend to look pretty literal as opposed to cleverly sardonic. Unless, I guess, you spend the whole day walking around with your tongue lodged in your cheek, but that might become a bit of a strain after an hour or so, and eating would be nigh impossible.)

Next, it has to be worn right, and this means, to continue the above point, not too literally. Blouses look best with jeans, as these keep a firm but friendly grip on the blouse to stop it from falling onto the stuffy side of the fence. You can just about get away with one with a pencil skirt but for the love of heaven, don't then get excited and slip on oversized fishnets and stilettos, as you yourself have now fallen on the "ironic" side of this apparently dichotomy-dividing fence. Short-sleeved blouses look nice with miniskirts or beneath short cotton dresses, but beware of tweeness, and a simple way to avoid this is to not get blouses with Peter Pan collars, which are slightly smaller than normal ones. A grown woman has no business wearing something with such a childish name (ref: kitten heel section in **Heels: the highs, the lows, and when fat is better than thin**).

But the biggest problem with the blouse is you. Well, your bust anyway. This is not a garment made for breasts, which is why for the past forty years the blouse's demographic tended to be the under-twelves; even librarians wear them only in films. It also explains why so many designers have become so fond of them, as many of them do seem to find body parts like hips and breasts intolerably intrusive on their Art. Few things make a woman's breasts look more like a threatening, clifflike single mass than a thin blouse stretched out over them with an almost visible grimace, buttons pulling apart in palpable pain. So in this case, the A cups win, and don't begrudge them too much because they deserve to get their kicks where they can. I mean, would you rather have a blouse or a bust? Two words: consolation prize.

Boots: the normal kind with a couple of variations

Remember when boots were just there to keep your legs warm? I know! Hilarious! Now they are so fashionable that magazines run solemn pieces every winter po-facedly advising which boot colors are in this season. You know that you are in Fashion-land when something is described as "wine-stained" as opposed to "purple." (Although here's a hint: unless you're in *The Rocky Horror Picture Show*, your boots should never be either.) It is stating the obvious somewhat (although this is a fashion book, so it would be downright illegal not to at some point) to elaborate on why boots are useful: they're flattering, they're warm, and they can be worn to work and to play. The downsides are that they can look totally awful and, somewhat impressively for a piece of footwear, they can make you feel fat.

At some point in the past five years manufacturers decided that the way to make high-heeled boots more fashionable and therefore more desirable was to make them narrower. Clothes designers, it hardly needs stating (although this is a fashion book, et cetera, and so forth), have been working this gimmick for years because items clearly made for thin people are somehow indicative of how up one's own market (as well as something else) one is. And this would be fine, albeit morally troubling, were it not for the fact that many customers discovered they couldn't get the wretched boots on their legs. No longer was just finding the correct size for one's foot the issue, now one had to bear in mind one's calf circumference, too. And for those of us who forget our damn PIN on a weekly basis, this can seem like a numerical demand too far.

Even when you've found a calf-tolerant boot brand, there are some rules. Absolutely never with bare legs unless you see the poster for *Pretty Woman* as your own personal *Vogue* magazine, in which case at least ignore that weird way Julia Roberts's top was pinned to her skirt—it was very annoying. Never out dancing unless you've always hoped for empirical evidence that your calves have sweat glands.

Boots in any color other than black, brown, and the occasional soft gray are illegal by order of the matter of taste, and patterned boots may result in custodial sentencing. Boots operate in a very similar vein to tights in that they should flatter your legs, keep them warm, and work with as many garments as possible; to splash them with bright colors and patterns pretty much decimates all of those requisites.

Because boots lengthen the leg automatically, you can get away with quite a small heel, even—gasp!—a kitten heel. For high heels, make sure you go chunky, unless you are still rocking *Pretty Woman* chic, though you may want to ask yourself whether you should take tips on something as important as footwear from a movie that advocated prostitution as a good career choice.

Biker boots are okay and rather fun to stomp around in, and are definitely to be preferred to Ugg-by-name-ugh-by-nature boots. Just don't wear them too literally, i.e., with a biker outfit, but rather with what proper fashion writers call "a soupçon of contrast," i.e., a posh dress or skirt and top, as opposed to a ripped kilt and safety pins.

As for cowboy boots, well. Although this book is in favor of using clothes to play dress-up and have a bit of fun in general, there are some looks which are forbidden unless they are an actual necessity. "Safari" is definitely up there in regard to all non-jungle-based activity, and skirts going by the somewhat un-PC name of "peasant" should not have their hems dragging along any kind of pavement. But number one is anything dubbed "cowboy." Jackets, shirts, and most of all boots are just about tolerable in a rodeo context, and that's merely out of respect for tradition coupled with a gracious tolerance for people who think standing around a dirt ring watching a man grip onto an angry bull constitutes a good night out. Because they make one's legs look thin and because they are associated with second-hand markets, they have become the favored footwear of posh girls. But, ladies, other things can slim the leg than some overly stitched boot, and the reason you always find them in markets is because they are rubbish and their owners have finally come to their senses and given them away. This latter point, incidentally, can be applied to overly floral dresses, mangy old fur, and beaten-up satchel bags (see **Vintage**). Men who favor cowboy boots believe that adding a couple of cheeky extra inches in height compensates for resembling some aging wannabe playboy strolling the beachfront on Capri. This assumption is mistaken. If you really do want to hike up your height, for heaven's sake just slip on an innocuous Chelsea or plain biker boot, or even a simple brogue with a subtle heel. Unless there really is a danger of your needing to round up the horses at a moment's notice, there is absolutely no excuse.

And as for pirate boots, my rising wave of despair somewhat swamps the necessary flame of outrage, leaving only mute distress.

Cardigans: a trend in action

The recent resurrection of the cardigan provides a useful illustration of the inner mechanics of a fashion trend.

Everyone knows the general trajectory: every six months the fashion magazines announce that a previously unthinkable look is just positively de rigueur this season. The public applauds and buyers eagerly flap their credit cards in the sales assistant's face. Six months later the style cognoscenti announce, with untroubled amnesia, that actually the look is hideous, and now it's all about some even more unlikely style.

Some say that this is merely the fashion industry's way of making people fork out their money twice a year on goods they heretofore never would have considered. Others claim that six months is the time it takes for the public to realize that their newly favored look of a tunic top over leggings, which once seemed ever so cutting edge, was actually sampled, then rejected, by Debbie Gibson twenty years ago. While both of these theories have a degree of merit, they are unnecessarily cynical. The truth is the public just likes new things. So just as, for a five-year-old girl, the once seemingly insurpassable appeal of Eskimo Barbie wanes with the arrival of Tahiti Barbie (and rightly so—the latter has hair down to her ankles), so those tunic dresses will soon lose their luster to those same girls several years on, thanks to overexposure, bad celebrities (see **Celebrities, and when bad ones happen to good fashion**), and, most important, the appearance of new clothes in the shops and on glossy magazine covers.

The cardigan is an interesting example, because here is a garment that was pretty much sartorial shorthand for mousy frumpishness that suddenly became the fash mags' latest sartorial pet. Not that this has ever prevented something from being dubbed a fashion trend, but there are several problems with the cardigan, hence its previous residency in fashion purdah. For a start, it is far fussier than a simple pullover in the way that it will always slip off one shoulder and hang in a niggling, uneven manner. Next, no matter how hard the sell made by the fashion dictators, there is no getting away from the fact that a cardigan would make even Serena Williams look a bit girlishly helpless, which not everyone sees as a boon. How very apt it was that the group that sang possibly the most simperingly twee song ever to appear in a half-decent film was called the Cardigans, known pretty much only for the grating song "Lovefool" from the otherwise pretty good *Romeo + Juliet* (points deducted for the stupid plus sign in the title). Finally, the age at which the cardigan slips from making a woman look sweetly feminine to decrepitly aged is very difficult to ascertain, and, thus, mistakes are often made.

To be fair, the cardigan wasn't an entirely outlandish garment to bring into the fashion fold. Proudly skinny ladies have long loved them because they keep their undernourished bodies warm, yet they also are slim-fitting, thereby showing off one's jutting shoulder blades and twiggish upper arms—hence their popularity with the likes of Coco Chanel and the ladies-who-(don't)-lunch. In terms of women's never-ending search for a garment that they can wear with a dress or jeans, it made for an understandable follower to the '80s shoulder-padded jacket and the '90s sporty, hooded top. Designers can get away with making expensive versions in cashmere and fiddly beading, while the mass market can knock out versions made so cheaply you can almost hear the gentle whimpers of sweatshop-bound children emanating from the stitches as you try them on. The cardigan fit in perfectly with the Mitford fashion trend in the early half of this decade. This did not, sadly, involve designers advising women to go to prison with their fascist husbands or to join the Communist party but rather to buy lots of tweed skirts, floral dresses, and, yes, cardigans, and generally look like they were on their way to buy a can of Carnation evaporated milk, ration book safely tucked inside a battered leather Mulberry handbag.

But a cardigan is not exactly a garment that puts one in the mood for breaking out the dancing shoes. Nor is it one that inspires much desire—it is a rare woman who gets too excited about buying just one cardigan, never mind four or five. They're quite a useful basic, yes, but unlike jeans, say, or a thin-knit T-shirt, there's only so much a designer can do with them; they can't be shaped to give you the bum of a California teenage surfing champion, and they can't be cut to give you Elle Macpherson's arms. The most a designer can do is just bead on another flower. Whoop-de-flipping-do. Occasionally you'll find either a super long or a cropped one, but these look more like the last desperate gasps of a garment struggling in the quicksand of ignominy than anything remotely useful or flattering.

Just as the cardigan was beginning to fade away, it saw a most unexpected development in its career: the men seized it for themselves. Well, I say the men did, but it was, of course, the menswear designers who then pushed it into the men's hands with a modicum of success. This was a clever ploy on the designers' part because a cardigan was probably not something a man already owned. He would have to—aha!—buy one. But the reason he didn't have one before is that the only man currently in the public eye who regularly wears a cardigan is Grampa on *The Simpsons*—who may spout the occasional memorable aperçu but does not, to be brutal, sport a look that most men, young or old, wish to emulate.

And that, of course, is its appeal. Because men's fashion still, incredibly, has to fight against weirdly conservative and often frankly homophobic prejudices, its braver souls often react rather like rebellious teenagers, opting for the most extreme and unlikely looks possible. This explains the endless carousel of neon clothes—patterned trousers—and garments so misguided they defy description (although here are three words: "Prada mohair leggings") that men's style magazines trot out every year. The eternal popularity of geek-chic clothing, popularized by labels such as Comme des Garçons, Jil Sander, and Prada, is very much part of this, as there is something so satisfyingly perverse about the idea of a designer anorak or a $1,000 patterned party shirt. Plus, seeing as men have yet to be convinced to spend a grand on a handbag in the way that women have, they must communicate their level of fashion awareness to fellow members of the in crowd with their clothes, and surely nothing says fashion in-ness better than a designer men's cardigan.

This does mean that the cardigan has a little more niche in the men's sector than it has in the women's. But at least it got an extended life and confirmed to designers that they might be able to conserve their precious brain cells and earn a few extra bucks simply by transferring clothes on the wane in the women's sector over to the men's, as they had done with skinny jeans. Best of all, it made a style icon out of a man who once perceptively proclaimed that the metric system was the tool of the devil.

Celebrities, and when bad ones happen to good fashion

Rarely has the phrase "making a deal with the devil" been more accurate than when describing the fashion world's alignment with celebrities. The appeal was always obvious and inevitable: a photo of Sarah Jessica Parker swinging around a Dior saddlebag gets far more press attention and ensuing sales than it does when carried by some unknown model on a catwalk. And you don't even have to convince the celebrities to wear anything: not long ago designers realized that just plopping some random TV stars into the front row of a show guarantees that the designer's name will appear in that week's issue of "Now!"/ "New!"/"Wow!"/"Who?" magazine that week, an ambition Cristóbal Balenciaga tragically died too early to achieve himself, and late at night, you can almost hear his spirit sobbing from beyond in regret.

With convenient synchronicity, celebrities realized that carrying the latest $3,000 bag got them extra magazine coverage, seeing as such shots proved an easy way for magazine editors to appease those pesky advertisers. Even more excitingly, some clever celebrities realized they could actually make a whole career out of this wheeze, with absolutely no particular ones coming libelously to mind. But because magazines propagated the idea that carrying a really expensive bag or wearing the latest Prada dress was somehow proof of the celebrity's inherent superiority over the rest of the world, as opposed to just being proof that they have a stylist, other celebrities from slightly further down the food chain began to get in on the act and this is when things became a lot more interesting.

Fashion is about image, from Dolce & Gabbana's molto sexy mentality to Marc Jacobs's aura of downtown cool, and it is this image that nudges customers to choose one over the other, depending on their ideal self-fantasy. The clothes are nearly irrelevant to the fantasy—that is created by advertising and celebrity association. Thus, Jennifer Lopez goes to a Dolce show, whereas Sofia Coppola is Marc Jacobs's front-row friend. So there is nothing like a celebrity at odds with the designer's carefully cultivated image daring to wear something from the collection to show just how fragile this system is and how utterly irrelevant it is to the general customer.

And for this reason, Z-list celebrities are the fashion customer's greatest friends. A Z-lister can be both the naked emperor and the wise little boy shouting about the nudity, giving an unexpectedly almost metaphysical element to a photo of, say, Jessica Simpson wearing a Prada dress. They show the reality of what the clothes are like, away from the image nonsense and prove that, while Cate Blanchett might look all glamorous and glacial, this has nothing to do with the dress she is wearing; it's because she is, duh, glamorous and glacial. Z-listers are the fashion litmus test because the clothes have to be not only good enough to look nice on normal women but so good that they can overcome the negative Z-lister association and, really, you shouldn't spend designer-level money on anything that offers less.

The most interesting example of bad celebrities destroying fashion items is that of Heather Mills, McCartney as was. The day after it was announced that this heartless woman was daring to get divorced from Saint Paul, she was photographed wearing, pretty much head to toe, clothes from her soon-to-be-former stepdaughter's collection. These included, most noticeably, over-the-knee boots, a look Stella had rather bravely been pushing for years. Some were confused by Heather's motives. Was she showing that, despite the increasingly acrimonious divorce, she was still a family woman, even if that family looked like they wanted to take out a contract on her life? Was she sending out an unlikely olive branch to Stella? Were the boots an ironic comment on the call girl accusations with which she had been lobbed? Was she just so damn cheap that, despite having access to wealth rivaling that of most African countries, she wore only clothes that she was presumably given for free? Or was it that she knew photographs of her wearing those clothes would cause far more damage to Stella than anything she could ever say in court? Frankly, it's almost enough to make you admire the woman.

Classics with a twist

Rhetorical questions are so annoying, aren't they? Nevertheless, it has to be asked, has this formula ever worked for anything?

A common irritant is boyish clothes that have been "girlified," such as dresses made from elongated hoodies or a pair of high-heeled sneakers, spawn of the devil if there ever was one. Kinda tough but still girlish in a Rizzo from *Grease* kinda way, is the intended message: wearyingly pointless and wincingly annoying.

With the exception of shorts, some miniskirts, and the occasional jacket, denim should be used only for jeans. There is something so redundantly gimmicky about dresses, long skirts, and trench coats made out of denim. "Yes, yes, well done," one yearns to say to the wearer of a denim coat, perhaps with a consoling pat on the arm. "You've taken a fabric usually used on trousers and used it for, yes, something else. Amazing."

A dress with a pattern usually reserved for home furnishings won't make you look like you are giving a cheeky nod to the brilliance of design in general; it will make you look like a sofa. And let's not even get started on three-quarter-length pants and miniskirts with cargo-pants-like side pockets, cropped pants and miniskirts being well-known garb for warfare. Obviously, wearing, say, plain black pants and turtlenecks is unremittingly boring, but a hee-hawing fashion gimmick is the sartorial equivalent of an embarrassing uncle doing a joke routine coined during the Crusades, in front of your friends, then punching them in the shoulder to ask if they got it.

Cleavage, and the plumbing of depths

Show me a woman with a good three inches of cleavage on display, and I'll show you a woman who, rightly or wrongly, has little faith in her powers of conversation. All fashion is, to a degree, some form of self-expression in that it gives onlookers an impression of your personality before you open your mouth. Some style choices, however, are there purely to head off the need to open one's mouth, simply because they come with such an immutable set of associations. Animal print is one such example (see **Animal print: when women roar**). Doc Martens boots on women is another. (Message: MAKE ASSUMPTIONS ABOUT MY SEXUALITY AND I'LL KICK YOU IN THE HEAD!) Cleavage takes this to a whole new level, because not only does it mitigate the need for conversation but any conversation attempted will be rendered pointless anyway since no one will be listening to it, because they're either (a) straight males and therefore rendered temporarily hypnotized—a cliché, yes, but sad and true; or (b) anyone else and thus are left shocked by the transparency of your tactics. There's nothing wrong with a woman embracing her sexual power, but when she hikes it up under everyone's nose with the desperation of a drunken aunt seizing the bar mitzvah mike for a quick impersonation of Chaka Khan, protests must be made.

Yes, you have breasts—congratulations. Whether squashing them together like two pigs fighting underneath a blanket shows them off to their best advantage is debatable. Whether it adds anything to your outfit is less so, because the answer is no, it doesn't. This is not to say you should button it up like Mother Superior, but, as Maria discovered in *The Sound of Music*, just a slight loosening of the habit is far more effective than a full-on vamp look, something the Baroness found out to her misfortune.

It's a common error among women. Just as you shouldn't spill out your life story on the first date (another frequent female mistake), so you shouldn't offer up the whole feast to the initial onlooker. After all, you want to be able to offer something later, don't you? For some women, getting out the cleavage is a Pavlovian response to the prospect of a big night out: they simply don't feel in the party mood unless they can keep hold of a couple of twenties and probably their mobile phone without the assistance of a handbag. But a big night out is precisely when you should tuck it away, simply because the potential for, as Janet Jackson might put it, "wardrobe malfunctions" is that much greater, so unless you want to look like Courtney Love in her '90s glory days, a bit of extra coverage is advisable.

A subtle V-neck is fine; a hint of more to come, courtesy of a wrap dress, grand; a full-on navel-plunging affair, unless you're in the Ziegfeld Follies, no. And anyway, do you really want to talk to men's flaking bald spots all night? Do you really think you have nothing more to offer than two pillows of fat squished together? And do you really want to attract the attentions of those men who are so easily hypnotized? Come on, girlfriend, raise the bar a little. True, Elizabeth Hurley made a career out of a cleavage-baring dress, but hers is a career some of us have never fully grasped anyway.

Clutch "bag"

With the noble exceptions of buttons and zips, always be wary of something that is named after its function. If the item in question was of any use, someone would have bothered to give it a proper name instead of just calling it by its verb. To whit, all a fly does is fly, and you can't do anything with a peel but peel it. The clutch confirms the truth of this age-old adage, and if you need further proof of this accessory's utter redundancy, the verb is not even a particularly nice one. Clutching on for dear life, clutching at straws—both perfectly acceptable phrases, yes, but hardly ones redolent of aspirational glamour or, in fact, any positive qualities at all.

The clutch has somehow managed to lay claim to being a member of the bag family, despite failing to fulfill what most would consider to be the two most basic requirements of a bag:

You cannot fit anything in it, and it is a complete pain to carry around.

This issue of bags at parties is utterly tedious because of the gaping canyon between pretty and practical. But a bag the size of a checkbook really won't help anyone strike a balance across that lacuna. With its faux suggestions of vintageness and its lack of strap, thereby not detracting from your exciting bare-shoulders action, the clutch has, with its wily, um, clutches, convinced female wedding guests around the world that it is the bag *de soirée du choix*. But look, at a party you actually do need to carry around quite a bit because, aside from the usual phone-keys-purse nexus, you will in all likelihood want to chuck in some makeup, a compact for occasional front teeth observation, and maybe an emergency bottle of water, absolutely none of which will fit into your clutch, and you'll find yourself actually wasting brain cells before the party by considering phrases like "Shall I sacrifice the crème blush for the lip gloss?" and "Maybe if I remove the cigarettes from the box they'll take up less room." (They will, but they'll all get crushed, and you'll never fully get all those flakes of dried nicotine out of the lining.) Even more annoying is that you have to carry the stupid, bulging thing around all night, like a cat presenting a freshly killed baby robin.

The whole point of a bag is to liberate your hands for important things like drinks, cigarettes, canapés, and flirtatious hand brushing. With the clutch, because you will only have one free hand, you end up having to do what is known in medical circles as the Party Multi-Finger Splay, holding the neck of your glass between your little and ring fingers, your phone between your ring and middle fingers and your cigarette between your first and middle fingers, which, as you light it, results in your spilling your drink down your cleavage.

And because you have to carry the clutch, you are guaranteed in your overexuberant party state to leave it somewhere, most probably under your chair or on that well-known black hole of ladies' accessories—the top of a toilet cistern.

So if you don't feel like ending the party in a drunken, hysterical frenzy, trying to find the damn clutch by calling your phone, only to be too drunk to remember your number, just get a respectably sized smart bag with a pretty strap. Honestly, there is not a man in this land who has ever thought, "Yeah, I'd have taken her number, but she had this really annoying bag swinging around her shoulders," and if there is, well, thank your prudent stars you were saved from any further encounters with such an accessories tyrant.

Coats: stuck at the nexus between dull and stressful

Under normal circumstances, few things please the human species more than an accepted excuse to spend lots of money on a single indulgence. Hence the enthusiasm among certain men for five-figure-priced watches (it's, like, science and art in one, see?) and pretty much the entire home technology market. (You watch TV every day, right? So may as well make it a flat-screen, high-def one, and don't spare the bank account!)

Like bags and shoes, coats fall under this umbrella in that they are to be worn every day, need to be made relatively well to withstand the elements, and have to work with a wide variety of outfits. Yet because they lack the crucial toy element of accessories, they simply don't spark the same excitement. Moreover, coats do not telegraph their designer status like bags do, most coats not being laden with gold chains and garish patterns (and we'll return to the problem of those that are), so they don't even have the mitigating appeal of flash. Instead, one is left standing in the department store coat section, whirling in a sea of black and gray woolen winterwear, freighted with a mental list of a coat's practical requirements. You are already wearied by the prospect of having to find something you can bear to wear every day and, frankly, quite tempted to say bugger it to the whole enterprise in favor of a watery in-store cafeteria cappuccino and a quick flick through *Us Weekly*. But limpid caffeinated drinks will keep a lady warm for only so long, so it's back to the coat issue. Obviously, the ideal would be to have as many coats as possible—maybe even a different one for each outfit. But not all of us can be the queen, so you need a coat that works with the probable two basics in your wardrobe: smart work skirts and jeans.

Princess coats—knee-length coats with a double row of buttons down the front, usually with a high, nipped-in waist and a small collar—have proven surprisingly adept in this area, as they look pretty with dresses and skirts and are a fast route to feminizing your Saturday afternoon hangover outfit of jeans and sneakers. Unfortunately, they can make you look like you're wearing Bonpoint for adults and thus are a touch infantilizing. For want of a better description, the recently popular pouffed coats—like princess coats but with the bottom half puffing outwards in a gentle oval—work better in this respect, just because they look more cleverly made and thus a little less Playskool.

Trench coats, too, work with skirts and jeans, but they fail to fulfill pretty much every other coat requirement and are thus to be treated with skeptical caution (see **Trench coats**). Similarly, because you need to wear your coat not just often but in multiple scenerios, don't get a patterned one. Aside from the fact that you will be so sick to the back of your teeth by the pattern come February that your fillings will actually vibrate every time you look at it (see **Patterns—or test patterns?**), you won't be able to wear your coat with half your wardrobe—i.e., your patterned half—without resembling a human acid trip. Moreover, there is something a little too deliberately wacky about the patterned

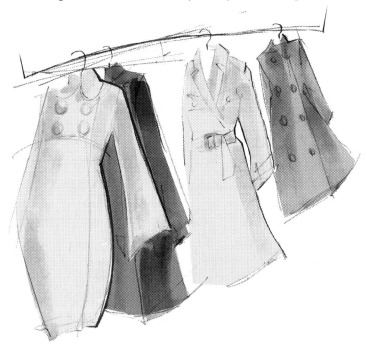

coat, particularly a winter coat, in its determined desire to announce one's cheerful nature to all and sundry. To be confronted with a red-and-pink-striped coat speckled with polka dots on the train home from work on a January evening is akin to being seized by the lapels by a chuckling fool desperate to recite to you Leno's "hilarious" routine from last night. For pretty much the same reason, brightly colored coats should also be worn stringently, so if you're buying only one coat, perhaps you should avoid those in Cheez Whiz orange.

Military-style coats can have a similarly wearying effect. On anyone who isn't actually in the military, they can make one look like the model of a modern major general in a local Gilbert & Sullivan revival, a Pete Doherty groupie, or—and this will unquestionably be the reference you get most from sniggerers— a member of the ROTC. Such negatives aside, the military coat does actually improve many outfits. Just as a sharp-tongued corporal whips a recalcitrant young scallywag into shape (editorial clarification to reader: all knowledge regarding the military in this book comes from *An Officer and a Gentleman* and *A Few Good Men*), so a strict military jacket pulls together a sloppy outfit, particularly the aforementioned hangover jeans uniform. Military coats often have belts, which is another boon because too many winter coats make one look even more lumpen than one tends to feel in the wintertime anyway. For this reason, A-line coats—occasionally called swing or trapeze cuts, presumably in an attempt to add a bit of all too rare circus fun to the subject of winter outerwear—can entirely disguise a body bloated with hearty food and winter inertia. However, you will be asked by uncomprehending male friends at least once a day whether you are pregnant, assuredly not a boost for a lady's sea-sonal affective disorder.

Similarly, full-length coats might provide the bodily cover-age factor with an added dose of drama, but sweep down the street in one on a dark winter's night and you will petrify onlook-ers convinced they are witnessing the resurrection of Jack the Ripper.

Ski jackets and parkas are the comfort food of the winter clothing world: their effect on your physical appearance is rarely beneficial, but they are what you retreat to when in that mood known to psychologists as "not giving a damn." For this reason, the reader is advised to own at least one of the above, even if the ski jacket will make you look like Kenny from *South Park*. The parka, meanwhile, with its waterproofed, coated sheen, comes in probably the only shade on the planet that doesn't look good on a single skin tone, but it allows you to wear your summer dresses in the winter, now worn with woolly tights, and, most important, will make you feel like you're walking around in a giant duvet. And, if we're being wholly honest here, that is pretty much what you're looking for from a coat in the first place.

Dates, and why they are the one event where you really don't need to worry about what you wear

Many movies contain essential human truths, but few have been better encapsulated in a single line of dialogue than one from *Clueless*. No, not the bit when Cher announces to her father that her day's achievement was that she "broke in my purple clogs" (although that can come in useful sometimes), but the moment when her quarry, Christian, leaves their video date abruptly, destroying her dreams of shucking off her virginity. "What's wrong with me?" she wails internally, throwing herself against the closing front door. "Did my hair go flat?" David O. Selznick died without ever helping to realize such a true piece of dialogue.

Of course, as all readers know, hair flatness was the least of the issues here. The fact that Christian was, in fact, gay may help to make this situation even more tragically familiar to female fashion followers. The point is that while Cher was fussing over the minutiae, Christian was looking at a much bigger picture, a picture Cher hadn't even considered.

Of course you want to look nice for your date. But do you know what looks best of all? You feeling comfortable, relaxed, and confident that you look good (and being the preferred sex). Yes, yes, this does all sound a bit cheerleaderish and fist-in-the-air but honestly, you could wear the world's shortest, slinkiest, sexiest dress, yet if you spend the whole evening tugging at your cleavage and pulling down the hem, you may as well have worn a burlap flipping sack for all the seduction you accomplish. So don't wear any stupid shoes you can't walk in and don't wear anything that will give you hypothermia; just stick with an old favorite that always makes you feel good and has garnered you compliments in the past. Honestly, he really, really doesn't mind if he's seen it before. Most boys don't notice that kind of thing, and, if they do, they don't care. They only have two jackets; who are they to judge? Generally, men take a Coldplay approach when it comes to women's outfits: if the overall melody is good, it doesn't matter whether the individual lyrics don't make the slightest dash of sense. A girl laughing and dancing and making sparkly conversation = attractive; a girl whining about being cold and insisting on getting a taxi to travel 200 yards = a colossal pain. The only exception to this rule is anything with writing, especially slogans, on it. Though obviously these should never be worn, period, unless you want your onlookers to feel like your chest is shouting at them, repeatedly. The other exception is anything too obviously slutty. Most guys are pretty mainstream and don't really want their girlfriends to look like the kinda lady who might nip off with their friends.

Sometimes you might want to play it extra safe, such as for a first date with someone you have fancied for ages and who took three years to understand that your getting drunk every time you saw him might suggest something other than alcoholic tendencies. For these crucial instances, you are advised to wear Clothes That Boys Get. The reader is encouraged to peruse the section pithily entitled **Get: fashion that girls do and boys don't** and do the opposite. So no empire lines, no voluminous dresses, no boatlike wedges, no smack-the-onlooker-in-the-face patterns, no three-quarter-length shorts, no smock dresses. I know—BORING. Fashion is about self-expression, so it seems a bit retro to subjugate the self for your date. But just as the female reader is not advised to spill out the gory details of past relationships or dabblings with mental illness on early dates, so it is a good idea to play it similarly safe in the clothes department. Leave him something to discover later, whether that be your lifelong mother issues or your penchant for sacklike tunic

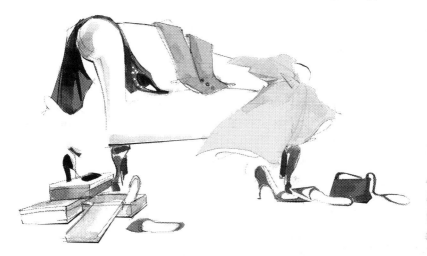

dresses. It doesn't hurt to pave an appeasing path up to your more exciting real personality. Hopefully you are making all this effort for someone who wants more than a weird mainstream female automaton, but if you don't and he's not, you'll spend the whole first date listening to dreary wisecracks about your much-cherished poodle skirt.

Here is what boys like: well-fitted skinny or bootcut jeans with a nice top, T-shirt, or V-neck sweater, maybe with boots over the jeans but ideally just some little heels or flats; a simple dress that nips in around your waist but is otherwise loose and feminine with (and you will begin to see a recurring theme in this list) a bit of a V-neck; a fitted dress of modest length—i.e., knee-length or just above—with a-bit-of-a-V-neck; a denim miniskirt with little heels or flats and a pretty (possibly beaded, possibly plain) top with a-bit-of-a-V-neck. Beginning to see the general point here, aren't you? Something pretty but unthreatening, something they could take home to meet their parents but that is still quite blatantly fanciable, something that is relatively modest but still suggests the possibility of a feminine body beneath. Yes, we are talking the sartorial embodiment of Cat Deeley. Or think of it this way: it's like leading a donkey to drink—you entice him with your wholesome nature but dangle a little bit of a carrot in front of his downy nose, hinting that there may be some joys to come besides water.

Meeting up with your girlfriends is actually a far more stressful fashion occasion, because they will notice the individual pieces, they will know what kind of look you're attempting here, and because none of them, presumably, will be mentally occupied by wondering whether you're going to put out, it will be hard to distract them with your fantastic body and gorgeous face. Hopefully, though, because they are your friends, they will take a tolerant attitude to any errors. If not, you may want to reconsider your wardrobe, not to mention your social circle.

Decade rehashing, and why designers live in the past

Gosh, it's exciting to work in fashion! Every season, one boards some magic time machine and emerges in a different time period! Wow! One year, we're all "very '50s," the next "it's all gone '70s" (this, it must be reiterated for emphasis, is obviously a reference to decades, not, heavens forfend, age). Partly, this is just a sign of laziness on the part of fashion journalists and designers. To the former, this kind of decade rehashing is just a sloppy and often historically inaccurate sort of shorthand for describing clothes when one's mental thesaurus runs dry. Hence, a dress with a tight waist is a sign that one has entered the '50s; the presence of a long skirt and floppy hat is a stronger indication than the unexpected reemergence of Jimmy Carter that we're back in the late '70s. Well, there are only so many times a person can write "high-waisted" or "long hems" before one eats one's elbow out of boredom.

To be fair to the journalists, designers are extremely fond of rolling back the years. From '60s shift dresses to '80s jumper dresses to '70s long dresses—all have been resurrected in modern times, and it is a rare year that doesn't have what is known in professional circles as "a bit of a flares moment." Some stand and cheer the designers' touch-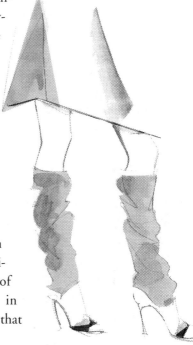ing respect for the past; everyone else, particularly those who lived through the decade being resurrected, cups their ears and detects the screech of a barrel scrape.

If, as is frequently claimed in those boring articles justifying "the point of fashion" or "the relevance of couture," a designer's job is to show us new ways to dress and, ergo, see ourselves, then wheeling out a bunch of mini-dresses, the subtle mechanics of which Twiggy instructed us in forty years ago, does indicate that someone, somewhere is falling down on the job. Possibly into a pile of cocaine in a nightclub in Soho, thereby stripping the brain of the cells responsible for "originality."

Moreover, there is something rather selfish about relying so heavily on the past. After all, what looks will we leave for our future descendants to copy? What on earth will TV bosses of the future be able to use to illustrate their I Love the Noughties programs? What, in short, will be our legacy? Hipster jeans? The thong? Ugg boots? Coinages to be proud of, one and all, and not, one could add, born from the catwalks. So remind me, what is the point of fashion again?

On the other hand, the only time this decade-revival shtick doesn't work is when something that is blatantly wrong is revived—flares, for example, spring readily to the mind. Otherwise, why shouldn't a nice flapper dress ('20s!) or cute tweed jacket ('40s!) be sported about town? It seems a little unjust that those born in the '70s, '80s, and '90s never get the chance to wear clothes with any form of structure purely owing to the misfortune of growing up in such a formless era.

If people can po-facedly claim that the Mitford sisters or Angie Bowie are this season's hottest trends, then wheeling out a time period doesn't seem that unreasonable. After all, fashion is literally just about dressing up. Dress yourself up like a communist or go for generic hippie—six of one, half dozen of the other, really.

And anyway, let's be a little sympathetic to the designers, because it's not like everyone doesn't idealize the past, in particular, the past of their childhood. This explains the current and seemingly never-ending '80s fashion revival because quite a few of the more popular designers today (Stella McCartney, Nicolas

Ghesquiere at Balenciaga) were kids in the '80s. It is a hard-proven fact that the most formative outfit in anyone's life is what their teenage baby-sitter wore when they were children. My God, did anything ever look so cool as what your sixteen-year-old neighbor wore as she sat on your sofa when your parents were out and talked on the phone to her boyfriend for three hours? Really, if designers seriously wanted to flog clothes faster, they would just get rid of the wan-faced models and hire a bunch of gum-chewing, pimply teenagers toting around their SAT-prep homework to walk the runways. Nothing like a Proustian moment to sell some ankle boots, as is proven by the fact that customers love this decade rehashing as much as designers do. If they didn't, the designers wouldn't do it. Pity the scraped barrel.

Dresses: God's gift to women

Yes, yes, we all know the theory that wearing trousers in the early twentieth century helped to liberate women from the shackles of male tyranny, et cetera, and so forth. Yet while this may have been a satisfying if symbolic triumph, one can't help but suspect that the words "Pyrrhic" and "victory" are more apt in this instance. For a start, liberate them to do what? Being able to dance the cancan without flashing their knickers? Climb a tree? Like, um, thanks.

Briefly, there is no garment more liberating to women than a dress. Except maybe a nice big hotel bathrobe, but we're not allowed to go to work in those yet. A good dress will never make you feel fat, it can be worn with flats or heels, and everybody can find a style that suits them—absolutely none of these statements can be applied to trousers with 100 percent certainty. I concede that some of the whaleboned dresses our grandmothers were fighting against in days of yore might have been a touch uncomfortable, but I haven't seen even a splinter of whalebone in H&M or Banana Republic recently, so I think it's safe to say we've left behind that millstone.

Trousers squeeze your waist, they squeeze your thighs, they often make your bum look the size of Ecuador, and they slip down ever so immodestly when you sit, and yes, I am including sainted jeans in all of these criticisms. Dresses do none of the above. With some judicious layering, you can wear a summer dress year-round, something you certainly cannot say about summer trousers, and the fact that you need to deal with only one garment in the morning is just the sartorial icing on this fashion gâteau.

Just as there is the old rule that the higher the hemline, the lower the heel, so there is a similar theory that says the higher the hemline, the longer the sleeves, perhaps merely to compensate in terms of flesh coverage. This isn't fail-safe, but long sleeves will make you feel a little less of a cliché than a minidress with spaghetti straps will, even if, to the male onlooker, the effect is pretty much the same, i.e., you're getting your thighs out. If you are going to go for a long-sleeved mini look, keep the dress fairly loose, like a tunic, unless your chosen Halloween costume this year is that of a Robert Palmer backup singer.

People get very stressed about which dress suits their shape; the fact is, you will, in all likelihood, figure this one out naturally. If you're a bit itchy around your waist and tummy area, you'll naturally gravitate toward a loose shift or tunic dress, and if you're rather fond of your curves, go for a dress that nips in at the waist, has cups at the bust, and falls flatteringly around the backside. The words "rocket" and "science" are not exactly springing to mind here. Anyone who makes out that buying a dress is any more complex than that is just trying to create a job for themselves. But one dress style that does need to be taken to task is the wrap. Much has been written by more manicured hands than my own about how brilliant this style is, how it (again, apparently) "liberated" women, how it suits everyone, and so on, and so on. Well, when anything is deemed to suit "everyone," you can pretty much disregard all the ensuing guff because that is clearly a load of rubbish (see also **Trench coats**). Nothing suits everyone, and wrap dresses definitely don't. If you have a curvy bust, a narrow waist, and a flattish stomach, well done; you have found your uniform. If you fall short in any of those departments, come and take a pew over on this side of the room. Moreover, its much-praised jersey fabric manages to be both unflatteringly clingy and immodestly loose, an impressive combination bettered only by Conan O'Brien's interviewing technique of being simultaneously greasily sycophantic and dismayingly crude. And finally, when the wind blows, well, suffice it to say you might be a little more liberated than expected. Whereas the joy of most dresses lies in their kindness to most body types or, at least, their ability to sculpt most body types into a flattering shape, the wrap is kind only to the chosen few and, if your body doesn't conform, it scoldingly emphasizes your alleged faults.

But wraps aside, dresses are the business, and they almost make up for periods, childbirth, and bad hair days. Pretty much in that order, in fact.

Drugs, the role thereof

"Whatever you said about [cocaine]," muses the middle-aged Park Avenue mother in Edward St. Aubyn's novella *Bad News*, "it wasn't fattening." Although that is definitely a major plus, fashion people could say a lot more about it, and they often do, but then it's amazing just how chatty two grams before midnight can make you.

Drugs are probably no more popular in the fashion world than they are on Wall Street, in the acting business, or in the music industry. Yet because the fashion world's image fits so nicely with so many of the clichés about drugs—the shallow glitziness, the surplus of cash, the not eating, the general talking of bollocks—it is now taken as a general assumption that if you work in fashion your septum must be just hanging in there, even if you are just the cupboard assistant and barely earn enough in a month to buy a bottle of Sudafed.

Yet there is no question that drugs are prevalent in fashion, pretty much for all of the reasons above. Heck, you'd really hope they are anyway: the thought that some of the things people come out with in this business, either in clothing or in their arrogant verbal hyperbole, are created in the cold light of sobriety is highly disturbing.

There is something about making a career out of what you did as a teenager—in this instance, going shopping and admiring yourself in the mirror—that does arguably arrest one's development, as many a rock star has proved in their time. Thus, there remains an attitude generally, but in the fashion world particularly, that getting hold of some drugs is proof of one's inherent coolness, even though any schlub with a spare $100 and access to a street corner could pull off that masterstroke. Anyway, the whole setup of the fashion industry today pretty much requires a constant supply of ready drugs. For a start, this is a business built on image. Before walking down the catwalk of a show, designers often put up little billboards backstage telling the models to look like fabulous, self-confident sex goddesses, even if it's 9 A.M. on a rainy morning in Milan and the models are all homesick, malnourished Russian sixteen-year-olds. "You are gorgeous and every man wants to fuck you!!!" a designer scrawled one season before his 11 A.M. show. Probably this would drive most women either to a pile of drugs to keep from laughing in his face, or screaming out the back door.

Even if he is on the verge of bankruptcy, a designer has to maintain an attitude of total confidence in order to give the brand its requisite aspirational desirability. Thus he has to say things like "Oh, you should have seen Jade and Kate on the nudist beach in Ibiza—it was just a riot" without throwing up his internal organs in self-disgust.

The publicists need something to cope with the pain of devoting their lives to the work of some screeching nobody with a personality disorder and to maintain total bubbliness in the face of fifteen-hour working days and being treated with, alternately, contempt and sycophancy by journalists, depending on whether their designer is having "a moment" or not.

Fashion journalists work in both fashion and the media, so if they somehow manage to avoid drugs in their career they probably aren't working very much.

The current fashion industry is about generating excitement

over things like handbags and pretending that you feel fabulous even if you're broke and haven't eaten since Wednesday or slept since Monday. Drugs are very useful in all these instances. Moreover, in the fashion world everyone is constantly on show and knows what everyone else is doing and, most important, their ranking in the industry. It is not beyond the realm of possibility that the only reason the antiquated system of fashion shows still exists is so that all the models, designers, publicists, and journalists get to spend four weeks together checking out not the clothes but each other (see **Fashion shows: Darwin in motion**). Cocaine may well have been created for moments such as these, to keep one's chin up, if nose down, when you see Anna Wintour clocking that you are in the eighth row. The nightly parties to celebrate such exciting events as a shop opening or a new perfume arriving at your nearest duty-free counter operate along similar lines.

Obviously, not everyone in fashion takes drugs. This is, although it is often forgotten, a billion-dollar business, which does suggest that someone out there is working on a Monday morning and not still monged out on Saturday night's ketamine binge. And as some aging designers have thoughtfully proven to the new generation, the sight of a sixty-five-year-old snorting coke, chuffing down sixty cigarettes a day, and burbling about the good old days when people knew how to show respect might well give him a certain image but not perhaps the kind that sells handbags.

Anyway, drugs are terribly bad for one's skin, and buying them is just shortsighted and shallow. Why spend a couple of hundred on white powder that will be gone by the morning when you can get something much more long-lasting and grati-fying, like a pair of Prada wedges? You see, not everyone in the business is superficial.

Ethnic clothes

Wonderfully useful word, "ethnic." India, China, Thailand, Togo—you name it, it's ethnic, which basically means "not Britain, America, Australia, and maybe France." In other words, it's not all that dissimilar to Archie Bunker's description of any-thing beyond his sofa as "a bit foreign" but with an added dose of faux hippie smugness.

From food to fashion, home décor to varieties of incense, if it looks a bit, well, foreign, and maybe smells a bit funny, it can be described as "ethnic."

Ethnic fashion is usually defined by an abundance of cheese-cloth, superfluous embroidery, and, if you're really going for it, gold trim. It tends to be particularly popular in delightfully pretty areas of town populated by large, well-appointed houses, three-wheeled strollers, and gourmet delicatessens, where one can find the most fabulous quinoa salad for just $15 a box. Fun-nily enough, what you rarely find in this type of neighborhood are any actually "ethnic" people, save those who clean the afore-mentioned well-appointed abodes. Well, maybe the clothes are there to compensate for their absence, as in pagan cultures in which dolls are dressed in the clothes of the dead to honor their absence. Or something.

Appreciating other cultures is always to be recommended.

And certainly there are many aspects to Eastern dress that one cannot but appreciate: it's often very pretty, ladies tend to be drawn to floaty fabrics, and, unless you've bought a belly dancer's costume, it generally gives good coverage.

The problem with this kind of fashion tourism is its underlying insinuation, which is generally about as subtle as a hot pink caftan top trimmed with little bells around the cuffs. There are three types of people who favor what they would describe as "the ethnic look": the liberal upper middle class, self-congratulatory travelers, and yoga teachers. All three use the clothes to send out the same message—namely, I am deeply spiritual, far above you with your West-o-centric lifestyle. Not so far above, mind, that I can resist shoving this belief in your face via my paisley caftan. Shanti, shanti.

I'm glad you had such an epiphanically life-changing experience in Jaipur/Marrakech/Ibiza—no, really, I am. But just as no one really wants to hear other people's holiday anecdotes, so they don't want to see them; wearing head-to-toe ethnic clothing is not very far from wearing your holiday pictures safety pinned about your person, and about as interesting. A small touch here and there—dangly silver earrings, say, or a floaty top with a pair of denim shorts, or some pretty flip-flops—fine; going for the full-on sequined Gandhi look when popping down to the organic market verges on an offensive costume. If we even get started on white people with dreadlocks, then this book will, I fear, descend into full-on expletives. Okay, fine, two words: sunburned scalp. You're feeling the spiritualism now, aren't you?

And to be honest, I'm not sure if buying embroidered tops from a boutique in the Hamptons, which itself bought them cheap as chips from a stallholder in Pushkar and then slapped on a 1,500 percent markup, is the best sign of one's affinity for another culture anyway. But, tempting as it is to suggest that the $300 for a pastel beach caftan might be better spent on a charity for that country, one doesn't want to be as smug as the ethnic lookers, so, with a pained sigh, let's just draw the curtain.

Exercise clothes: the new couture

This is a true story: because of a clerical error, I recently stayed at a ridiculously fashionable hotel in Beverly Hills. Wanting to take full advantage of this most unfortunate state of affairs, I sauntered on down to the pool in my favorite plain black bikini, a pair of simple black shorts, and some flip-flops, and ordered breakfast. From the general reaction, you'd have thought Mrs. Shrek had taken up residence, poolside. My first mistake was that, despite being female, I had ordered food. The other mistakes were almost as shameful: first, my bathing suit was notably lacking in Versace gold chains, Gucci military detailing (think Halle Berry in James Bond), Missoni tassels, and other similar ornaments that generally suggest one is more interested in letting others know that you spent over $400 on a bathing suit than in any actual swimming. And what was I thinking, going for French Connection shorts instead of a designer sarong, aka a long scarf that falls off every time you try to stand up, owing to scarves' generally being made to go around one's neck, not one's waist? That I had neglected to put on makeup—yes, makeup at 10 A.M. to, lest we forget, lie by the pool—was almost incidental.

Fine, this is a fairly extreme example, as examples from LA tend to be. But it is the magnification of a general truth: ever since the '80s, when exercise became fashionable, it was inevitable that its accoutrements and uniform would have to follow suit. Go to any yoga class and marvel at the predominance of cute little tank tops decorated with lotus flowers by Christy Turlington's nuala label and sexily low-slung velour trousers. There are even trends regarding yoga mats (pink is very passé; it's all about natural fibers now, or at least Stella McCartney's dusty-rose version for Adidas), just as the Indian yogis always hoped for. Go to a gym and delight in all the increasingly suited-up sneakers that look like they were invented to assist the wearer on a moon voyage, as opposed to managing thirty minutes on the step machine. Inevitably, it is the trendiest sports—surfing, skiing, and yoga—that have the strictest and snobbiest rules regarding fashion, finding every year with a new rubric. The "what to wear on the slopes" feature is now an annual staple in fashion magazines.

On one level, I cannot but applaud this trend toward making any actual exercise irrelevant. And there is something very pleasing about the idea of self-described gym fans shopping for ever more expensive exercise outfits as a way to avoid getting on the treadmill. Well done, O athletic ones—so glad you have come round to the general view at last.

But after seeing one too many photos of Kate Moss on the slopes with her baby daughter, the former in a giant fur hat, the latter in Dior Baby ski boots, well, even the most exercise-phobic lady can find herself thinking wistfully back to the days when one could wear paint-stained tank tops and sagging shorts to the gym instead of worrying whether retro Kappa or futuristic Nike was the look that week. Now the only thing you can wear a paint-stained tank top to do is paint your front room. Everyone knows what body fascists personal trainers and gym receptionists can be. Well, take that snootiness and imagine it in regard to gym outfits and you've got a whole new level of *Mean Girls* bullying going down at your local yoga center.

Still, it's always nice to see that even supermodels find exercise a bit of a bore and seem only to drag their skinny butts out there these days to show that they, too, have, like, totally got into this new layering of tank-tops shtick.

Fashion shows: Darwin in motion

Some people find that looking up at the vast black sky peppered with stars gives them a vertiginous epiphany about their own smallness in the great scheme of things. These people have clearly never been to a fashion show.

There is a general belief that fashion shows are somehow glamorous affairs. It's an idea perpetuated mainly by films (see **Films about fashion, and why they are all (mainly) rubbish**), although seeing as movies about, say, London seem to think that the only habitable area is Notting Hill and that Dick Van Dyke wasn't actually that far off on the ol' accent does suggest that perhaps we shouldn't take too many lessons from the silver screen.

In truth, fashion shows are brutally cruel affairs. They have nothing to do with the clothes: if they were about fashion, designers could just put their collections on the Internet instead of making the entire industry schlep around to New York, London, Milan, and Paris twice a year, save everyone a lot of money, and reduce their carbon footprints.

The real reason fashion shows exist is to teach everyone in the business their place. For designers, pecking order emerges from where on the schedule the fashion council puts their show: if it's at, say, 9 A.M., they are generally pretty much down there with Wal-Mart in terms of fashion credibility. Sometimes, though, this works in reverse, and occasionally very important shows get the hated early morning slot, a clever ploy on the part of the schedulers to get hungover journalists out of bed and away from their room service. How many people come to the show and who they are is also indicative of a designer's caste. Anna (Wintour, US *Vogue*), Cathy (Horyn, *New York Times*), Suzy (Menkes, *International Herald Tribune*), Alexandra (Shulman, UK *Vogue*), Glenda (Bailey, US *Harper's Bazaar*), Carine (Roitfeld, French *Vogue*), Carla and Anna (Sozzani and Piaggi, Italian *Vogue*), and Katie (Grand, general fashion supremo) are pretty much the designer's dream front-row guests. A bunch of friends from fashion college and his mother are, rather heartlessly, not. The irony is that attendance is generally dictated by advertising (see **Advertising: how it spins the fashion axis**), in that if a designer advertises in a publication, that editor is forced to go to the show. Yet the only way designers can afford to advertise is if they become successful, and the only way they can do that is to catch the eye of one of the above editors. Parsing that vicious circle could burst a blood vessel in a gentler mind.

It's the journalists who get the harshest lessons, repeatedly, for four weeks, twice a year. There are few things that will teach you your place in the universe more swiftly than arriving at the entrance to the show, all decked out in the latest Alaia, proving to your colleagues that, yes, you know how to spend money, only for the eagerly awaiting paparazzi to lower their cameras as one in disappointment. This is usually followed by their shouting at you to get out of the way because you are standing in front of that hot girl who was in *Aquaman 3—The Fish Is Back*.

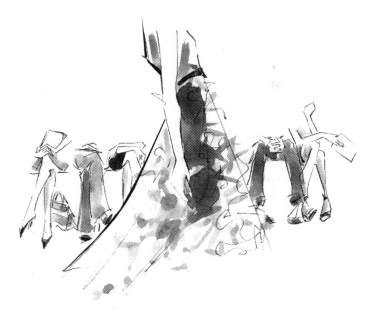

Then you're in the tent. Yes, a tent. It is a rare fashion show that is in a posh salon: more often they're held in a giant wedding-marquee-style tent or some horrible dark basement or, if the designer is just terribly "edgy," in a cold warehouse in the middle of pig-all nowhere, ideally in the dead of night and the depths of winter. You look at your ticket, and this is when the proper humiliation starts. What seat you've been given by the publicist is a very public statement of your importance or otherwise in the industry. The processes by which this is decided are mysterious. Fashion show seating arrangements are quite possibly one of the first matters of discussion at the Bilderberg Group conferences. Henry Kissinger, in particular, is said to be a real tyrant about them.

If you're in the front row, you must sit down immediately so that as many people as possible can see your positioning. Second and third row are bearable, as long as none of your colleagues are in front. Anywhere back from that and you have been well and truly cast out of paradise. Several options now await you. You can sit and grouse to everyone around you about how at every other show you were in the second row, the seating this time is crazy, I mean, look who's in third over there, I mean, they must have had the work-experience girl do the seating this time, well, you won't be using any of the designer's clothes in your magazine this season, that's for sure.

Or you can cover up the number on your ticket and take a sly seat in the second row in the hope that its rightful owner doesn't turn up.

Or you can force a grin, lump it, and sit in your seat, and pretend you are above it all.

Or you can do what you really want to do and yell at the

publicist like a banshee, but you do have to weigh up the pros and cons on this option. On the plus side, it is rather satisfying and will probably get you a better seat next time around, if not now. On the downside, it can be rather humiliating to hear yourself having a public temper tantrum about a chair.

Worst of all is the dreaded "ST" on your ticket. This means "standing," as in, that's what you'll be doing at the back, as in, you're not even worthy of any chair, no, not even in the eighth row. You have absolutely no choice at this point but to leave the show and pretend you have been urgently called into the office.

So now you're in your seat at the precise moment the show is supposed to start, and you wait. And wait. And wait. And wait. When you get, say, a theater or movie ticket, the start time on the little slip of paper does tend to be exactly when your entertainment commences. The time on a fashion show ticket has absolutely no bearing on when the show will start, except maybe being within a general two-hour estimation. No one has yet come up with a satisfactory explanation of why this is. Yes, some people will make annoying noises about how it takes a while to get the models from show to show and then make them up in time and blah, blah, blah. But considering that fashion shows have been taking place for about a hundred years, you'd think that designers and schedulers would have realized this by now and come up with a realistic running time instead of telling audiences to get to a "3 P.M." show only to then make them wait, chewing on their knuckles with boredom, for the show's actual start at 4:39. The truth is, it is just another example of the kind of teenage attitude that dominates the industry (see **Drugs, the role thereof**), allowing that being late is somehow cool: the designer is basically saying my time is more valuable than yours, and I am just much busier than you, you lowly layabouts.

Sometimes, though, the show is running late because of a celebrity, and this is pretty much the final nail in the journalist's ego's coffin.

Fashion journalists like to think that they are the most important people at the show, and they sit on the sidelines like Roman emperors, while the designer waits with bated breath to see if their manicured thumbs will point up or down. They are disabused of this illusion when they are kept waiting for two hours (or have we already mentioned this?) because front-row guest Tori Spelling hasn't arrived yet. The fact is, a paparazzi photo of a celebrity in the front row will do more for a designer's career than a front-page headline proclaiming his brilliance. The word "irrelevant" haunts the journalist on many dark nights of the soul.

And then, at last, the show starts. And then it's over. Yes, all that fuss for a seven-minute event. In order to reconfirm one's sense of unimportance, the designer will then come out and give personal waves to the carefully chosen few. Then it's the mass exodus, with everyone who was so desperate to get in and be given their important seat now suddenly so consumed with desperation to leave you'd think polonium had been discovered on the premises. If you are important, you will have either a bouncer (for celebrities) or a dedicated minion (for fashion editors) to plow a path for you through the crowds to ease your exit. Everyone else will have to fight their own battle. But hurry! There's no time to waste! The next show starts in twenty minutes, you know!

Fashionspeak

The poet Joseph Parisi once said, "Among the foremost reposi-
tories of demented language today are fashion magazines, art
journals and the back covers of poetry books." One can see
where he's coming from, but Parisi rather overestimates the linguistic capabilities of art criticism and poetry publishing.
Although both of those industries, particularly the former, rely
heavily on the parlance of nonsense in order to maintain their
elitist images, neither has managed to coin a lingua quite so
unfrank(a) and so un-Saussureanly disconnected from the real
world as fashionspeak. After all, this is an industry that runs on
a schedule predicated on some previously unknown timescale
that consists of only two seasons a year, called "autumn/winter"
and "spring/summer." Latinate in origin, Chinese in incompre-
hensibility, fashionspeak is a lot like an onion in that it contains
many layers that merely conceal more layers; it can cause tears
of frustration, and it just keeps repeating on you no matter how
grimly you swallowed it the last time.

But before you stroll down the easy path of mockery, take
pause and consider the actually fairly justifiable reasons for its
existence. For a start, trends are, as they say, circular in nature
(fashionspeak for "frequently regurgitated"), and there are only
so many times a person can repeat "pencil skirts are back" before
the will to live seeps from the saggy, despairing soul. So thank
God for coinages, such as "it's all about the '50s" (see **Decade
rehashing, and why designers live in the past**) and "the sexy
secretary is huge this season," no matter how nonsensical they
may well be out of context.

Next, the majority of fashion journalists are not specifically trained in their field, unless a lifetime of shopping counts. And so, not entirely unlike the psychotic government officials from Orwell's apocalyptic vision of the future in *1984*, they rely on an empty lingo to create a veneer of professional credibility. But most of all, they're trying for a bit of variety instead of just repeating what they really mean, which is "I quite like these clothes; they would look good on me," which admittedly might have a kind of novel honesty to it but would get a bit tedious repeated eight times a day, every day, for fifty years.

Finally, fashion shows run very, very late. On a typical fashion-week day, the poor, huddled masses will spend approximately eight hours and forty-seven minutes gazing into dead space, tapping their pens against their carefully chosen Smythson notebooks, waiting for a wretched show to begin. Thus, a lady or gent has a lot of time to think deep thoughts, such as exciting new synonyms for words like "beige" and "good" in the same space of time in which they could probably find the cure for cancer. "Homage" is probably the most well known bit of fashionspeak. A conveniently trussed-up word for "blatant copy," it can be used without the niggling fear of litigation, and it has a soothing sheen of intellectualism, suggesting that the designer spent long, noble hours in some dusty library, studying the technique of his forebears and then respectfully weaving it into his own work, as opposed to desperate plagiarism due to a dearth of new ideas. So, for example: "Marc Jacobs's homage to Courrèges was perhaps a little over-literal." Thus, it becomes a criticism in a compliment inside a totally daft remark, showing the kind of linguistic ingenuity that would make Derrida bow down in respectful awe.

Closely related is "inspiration," used to denote the desperate recourse of a designer who has still not come up with any ideas two weeks before the collection is due. Off they hie hence to their teenage music obsession, a cinematic hero of old currently enjoying a bit of a renaissance or a painting in some heavily publicized exhibition at their local museum and then copy the bejeesus out of it. As in "Golly, Gucci really got a lot of inspiration from David Bowie this season."

"Channel" is another useful term here. It sounds like a term a TV psychic might use when claiming an ability to resurrect the spirit of a dead person through their body, and, actually, it does mean something like that. In the fashion world, "to channel" means that one is deliberately styling oneself to look like someone else, usually a dead former style icon, as in "You might wonder why I am wearing a multicolored chiffon caftan and oversized sunglasses in London in November, but I am totally channeling Talitha Getty this season."

Fashionspeak is essentially about giving an aura of gravity to what is undeniably a frivolous pursuit. "Invest" is one such example in that it suggests that getting another Betsey Johnson party dress is on a par with prudently buying stocks, as in "Yes, that $600 dress is a bit on the pricey side but, you know, it will be a great investment." Similarly, "archive"—or "put into storage" to most people—is a more advanced example and, as such, is used mainly by the well-practiced fashion linguists, i.e., the American fashion press and models. It gloriously conflates one's wardrobe with, say, a library of medieval manuscripts, as in "All of my wrap dresses have gone out of style this season, so I'll archive them."

"This season's essential" or "must have" is the bass line of fashion writing. And really, one's only response can be, bossy, bossy, bossy! Fashion people love a good imperative, maybe because this kind of fearsomely brook-no-argument tone helps to trample over any bleating objections or queries as to why a $3,000 handbag with a handle made from the bone of a woolly mammoth and stitching from the hair of an albino virgin is apparently as necessary to someone's life as water. But there is some literal truth in the phrase, as it is usually used in connection to this season's most expensive accessory by a company which has spent a particularly large wad on advertising, the sort of advertising a magazine must, ahem, have.

Another good one is "experimentation is key." This is the telltale phrase that the designer or fashion journalist hasn't a freaking clue or is hedging some unlikely bets, as in "Should you have a short waist but a long torso, you should wear bias-cut skirts, but experimentation is key" and "This season's de rigueur shade of bright mandarin looks just great against most complexions, but experimentation is key." As practice, perhaps try using this handy phrase in all walks of life, not just fashion, e.g., "Honey, do you know how on earth you fill out these wretched tax forms?" "Hey, experimentation is key!"

But it is in descriptions of collections that the essentially euphemistic nature of fashionspeak comes into its own. To describe a collection as "very editorial" means that, as the designer appears to have taken the gimp from *Pulp Fiction* as his style inspiration this season, the clothes could only work in some edgy fashion shoot and won't ever see the light of production. Conversely, "very commercial" means the clothes are very boring and all those beige trousers and black coats will sell by the bucketful in (sniff) Middle America.

The various terms of approval for a collection are plentiful, reflecting the essentially positive nature of fashion journalism (see **Advertising: how it spins the fashion axis**). "Spot-on," for example, is "good" but with a gratifyingly bossy ring. "Modern" means "a bit different from last season"; ditto for "vibrant," which is basically "modern" but with extra colors and maybe a frill, and ditto for "fresh," which is exactly the same, except perhaps with particularly young models in the show. "Witty" is a polite word for "so gimmicky even Andre 3000 would balk at wearing it," as in "Moschino's take on French coquettes, replete with striped T-shirts, petticoats, and berets, was wonderfully witty." "Daring" is the synonym for "unwearable," as in "a certain British designer's collection of balloon clothes was excitingly daring." "Romantic," and occasionally "whimsical," can be read as "simperingly floral." All of these terms are used with notable frequency by the American fashion press in particular, who perhaps have starved themselves to such an extent that the oxygen is no longer reaching the brain area, thereby disturbing their ability to use the English language anymore.

Colors allow designers and fashion writers to indulge their thwarted teenage poetic longings. "Taupe," "camel," "putty," "oatmeal," "biscuit," "sand," and "nude" are all beige; "ivory," "snow," "virginal," and "oyster" are white; "cherry blossom," "blush," and "flush" are all pink. Jewels are always useful, as in "emerald" for green or "sapphire" for blue, although in the latter instance, should you be going for a more cerebral element, it is better to say "very Yves Klein." Perhaps most poetically, "cappuccino" is better known to the masses as pale brown. Cruder mouths might refer to this kind of adjectivalizing as gold-plating some dung, but as long as the dung is described as "mocha," everyone will be happy. "Dove gray" is another ersatz reference point, even though doves are generally considered to be white. But maybe a lot of fashion people are just color-blind, which would, at least, explain the enduring appeal of Pucci.

There is even a word for the use of color, period. "Pop" basically means some color in an otherwise dull outfit, as in "Sharon Stone livened up her LBD (little black dress) with a pop of color from her red belt." "Shot through" is another popular one, adding a bit of dynamism to what is otherwise an immobile piece of clothing, e.g., "Dolce & Gabbana's black miniskirts were shot through with a hint of silver."

Textures, too, come in for some gold-plating treatment. "Butter-soft" is a particularly popular one at the moment. It is used only in regard to leather, which in reality tends to be more smooth than soft and not generally reminiscent of a melting dairy product.

Festivals, and why they're a bit like being pregnant

There was a time when a person at a music festival was considered quite the definition of high-maintenance chic if they put their dog on a leash instead of favoring the more traditional muddy-string method.

Now that festivals have been taken over by musicians' fashion model girlfriends and tickets are so expensive they can be bought only by the upper middle classes, music festivals have become a veritable fashion industry in themselves, from Coachella to Lilith Fair to South by Southwest. Every year, the fashion press greets the advent of summer with the traditional "what to wear at a festival" feature, in which helpful suggestions like "go for the layered look" tend to be made, usually illustrated with a Marc by Marc Jacobs parka ($360 for you, good madam) and a Sonia Rykiel jumper dress ($450, thanks).

In the main, though, clothes at festivals haven't changed that much—it's just that the extremes have become more marked. So those who look effortlessly fabulous on a daily basis look annoyingly fabulous sloshing about in the mud decked out in several cropped sweaters they picked up in the West Village, layers of Victorian slips they found in some vintage store, and a fabulous pair of Wellingtons that make their legs look even thinner than usual. The rest of us, however, spend seventy-two hours in some badly fitted jeans, our older brother's discarded Gap hoodies, and sneakers that prove one needn't go to war to get a tasty dose of trench foot. In this way, festival dressing has become a bit like maternity wear in that we are now told that it's all gone very fashion and we have to wear 7 For All Mankind maternity jeans and Juicy Couture tunic tops in order to be accepted by our fellow sufferers. Such diktats may well be embraced by those to whom such diligence comes naturally. The remaining 99.99 percent of the population, however, happily embrace the occasion as an excuse to dress how, secretly, we all occasionally wish we could year-round: like homeless slobs for whom the words "waistband," "high heel," and "color coordination" have as much relevance to life as a "juice fast."

In point of fact, being at a festival has many similarities with being pregnant: you're physically uncomfortable, you're surrounded by people who are younger, thinner, and more energetic than you, and you feel like you're spending your life looking for a bathroom. But, as with pregnancy, there is generally a happy ending. For a start, festivals are fun, but only—and I realize this is somewhat maverick advice from a fashion book—if you totally give up all thoughts of fashion. The only important things to ask yourself when robing yourself for a day at a festival are: Will this keep me warm? Will this keep me dry? Will this keep me protected in the porta-potty (i.e., no flip-flops)? Thus, you are advised to model yourself on one of the magic mushrooms you will be offered as soon as you arrive by decking yourself in a luminous waterproof poncho (making it easier for your friends to find you) and wearing sludge-colored trousers to help the mud blend in that little bit easier. Don't wear anything knitted, as you will smell like a mangy cat when it—as it always will—rains. You should take one tip from your more fashion-fabulous fellow attendees: Wellingtons are strongly advised, if only because they'll make it easier to kick people out of the way in the line for a baked potato. Yes, you will look a complete fool, but come three in the morning, while the more delicate flowers are shivering in their vintage slip dresses, you can snigger up your chunky parka sleeve and will be able to carry on regardless, accruing all sorts of anecdotes, the majority of which will probably involve Nick Cave. And don't be cowed by the celebrities; they all get to stay in the VIP area, which probably has running hot water, central heating, walk-in wardrobes, and, for all I know, personal stylists on tap. After all, even Kate Moss could catch trench foot. Nick Cave, however, is probably superhuman.

Films about fashion, and why they are all (mainly) rubbish

Funny thing, this issue about fashion in movies. Seeing as the former is an industry based on visuals, you'd think that there would be few other subjects that would lend themselves so easily to being depicted on screen. However—from *Designing Woman* to *Funny Face* to *Prêt-à-Porter* to *The Devil Wears Prada*—there has yet to be a movie about the fashion business that is less shallow than the world it purports to cleverly depict and sardonically critique, simply because such films rely more strongly on the rehashing of creaky clichés than a whole week's worth of Fox TV sitcoms. Let's see, there's the harridan of a boss, bitchy journalists who never eat and seem able to afford Chanel couture despite earning about $6 a day, sleazy photographers, queenly designers, and expensive freebies raining down like wedding confetti. Honestly, at least you could do your subject matter the honor of making up some jokes that postdate World War II. Even Rodney Dangerfield updated his set every couple of decades. Surely it couldn't be that the filmmakers themselves get so distracted by all the glitz and pomp they're allegedly satirizing that their brains are rendered incapable of finding new jokes or penetrating the industry's surface?

God knows the fashion world has its absurdities, and it is a lot easier to send up than, say, peacekeeping missions in the Middle East. So, yes, showing a big editorial meeting in which the topic up for solemn discussion is whether one should do a double-paged spread of red shoes or blue hats might have some appeal for a filmmaker. But that is what these magazines are about, as anyone who opened one could see: it's not necessarily any more surreal than showing the editorial meeting of a car magazine, say, in which the hot topic for discussion is whether a man should go for bucket seats or leather upholstery. The word "illuminating" is not generally one that comes to mind when watching a movie about the fashion business.

Aside from the staleness of the jokes, it's the unsubtle underlying message that grates. Movies about fashion always mock or punish the women who work—very successfully, incidentally—in an industry they enjoy. In *The Devil Wears Prada*, for example, the Anna Wintour–ish magazine editor might be the most powerful woman in fashion, but her husband leaves her because, as far as can be ascertained, she had the temerity to be late for dinner occasionally owing to work obligations. In an almost identical plot in *Sex and the City*, Carrie's magazine editor is often spotted having lonely solo lunches or hiding shyly in the corners at parties, and the only human relationship in her life is with a man whom she has to share with another, younger woman. And it's not that they work in just any industry but in one that is dominated by other females. Oooh, scary! It's like some sci-fi dystopian nightmare! Thus, fashion magazine employees are invariably depicted as childish, narcissistic bitches. See what happens when you let the silly billies work together in a closed environment? Give them a second and they'll start lobbing maxi-pads at each other. Hence the inevitable character of the friendly, usually gay, man in the office, usually working as the art director or something vaguely masculine. Sure, he might have chosen to work in fashion but at least he's not riddled with estrogen.

Career women rarely come off well in movies anyway:

fooling around with a generic leading man is still widely viewed as the happiest ending; a promotion or deal clinch is merely a gloss on an otherwise lonely life spent eating TV dinners in front of *Friends*. But because the fashion industry is generally seen as pretty silly, filmmakers treating the subject can get away with more. Thus, a woman who seriously devotes her life to it, instead of acting all Sandra Bullock–ishly kooky, charming every passing man, can more easily be depicted as being blind to the important things in life and an all-around self-deluding bitch.

As with all the guff about how fashion surfs on a wave of cocaine, fashion is a multibillion-dollar industry, and it would be awfully hard to keep that afloat if its movers and shakers sat around all day fretting about the high sugar content in grapes, pausing only to stab one another in the back.

This is neither a plea for fashion to be taken more seriously nor even a complaint about Hollywood's injustice to fashion assistants, which, as causes go, is probably not up there with calls for racial tolerance. But fashion on many levels magnifies female issues in popular culture, from the exaggerated body fascism in the industry to its interest in self-expression through physical appearance. So films' wholesale dismissal of women who work in fashion highlights the very outdated misogyny one still sees in pop culture not only toward successful women but also toward women doing something that has shockingly nothing to do with men.

The fact that these films and TV shows don't come within ten miles of anything approaching accuracy is a secondary niggle. Still, skinny women wearing Roland Mouret dresses sniping at each other in white-walled offices makes for a better scene than, say, a stylist's assistant packing up boxes of clothes in the fashion cupboard or a woman—gasp!—finding personal fulfillment in her job. And that's the main thing, right?

Flat boots

There are undoubted military associations to the flat boot, particularly fascist ones if yours are, as they should be, long and narrow. But as long as your boots are not too (a) shiny; (b) clunky; and (c) prone to being kicked in other people's faces, it's unlikely that anyone will confuse you with Goebbels. As much as everyone delights in reeling back in horror when an attention-seeking designer claims to have found inspiration in, say, the homeless (ah-Gallianochoo!), in truth, flat boot designers are not, by and large, trying to raise the specter of Göring. There's just not that much money in that look these days, what with the National Front not having quite made the cover of *Vogue*.

Flat boots are marvelous because they have all the comforts of normal flats yet give your legs more definition. And they are far better to be worn over jeans than are high-heeled boots, which just make everyone look like prance-prance-prancing My Little Ponies. Some women fear that these boots will make them look like members of a marching band, but as long as you don't pair them with any red items that have brass buttons you should be fine. And don't march.

Yet it's not all good. When a designer knocks out the flat boot he is more often than not evoking what he calls "the equestrian look." Designers love the equestrian look, not because they idolize jockey Frankie Dettori (although that man is just fabulous at keeping his weight down) but because they associate it with the upper classes. Unlike a lot of people, when designers talk about the upper classes, they don't mean the unattractive, dull-witted, incestuous sorts you'd find in an Evelyn Waugh novel, but rather the breezy, arrogant types Helena Bonham Carter used to play in movies before she stopped brushing her hair. This is mainly because they think these are the people who can afford their clothes, when in fact, as pretty much everyone else knows, these old-school aristos tend to be utterly broke, not having worked for the past thousand years and spending the inheritance on buying heroin and having the roof fixed.

Flat boots with superfluous buckles and buttons down the side are classic examples of the equestrian look.

Another kind of flat boot that has equally odd and, one would have thought, anachronistic associations is the chunky flat boot. The Ugg, the extra-wide-mouthed Wellington, and anything fur-lined fall into this category because they are deliberately capacious enough to make the calf look as thin as possible, like a little toothpick popping out of a sickly cocktail. As tactics go, it isn't subtle, but it is very effective. However, once you notice that it makes you look like you're about to be sent to sleep with the fishes, it is hard to stick with it.

Flat boots should, by rights, be one of the most basic things in your wardrobe. It's when people start trying to [insert waving jazz hands movement here] liven them up a bit with buckles and buttons and fur that they became utterly ridiculous (see **Classics with a twist**). Granted, Ugg boots are ever so cozy, but I'm afraid they are another example of a fashion item that has been ruined by bad celebrity association (see **Celebrities, and when bad ones happen to good fashion**). And as for men wearing Uggs, there should be a law. Literally, a law.

Fur: bad

Let's make this a quick one, shall we? Unless you are an Eskimo or maybe following the route of the Trans-Siberian Railway on foot in January, there is no excuse for wearing fur, not now, not ever. Look, you know the facts, and if you don't, here they are summed up in speed-readable form: electrocution, anal probes, drowning, strangulation, tiny coops, orphans, skinned fetuses, forced abortions, blinding, beating, and if anyone tells you that their pelt is the "by-product" of the meat industry, five out of ten times they're wrong, and four out of ten times they're lying, and the remaining one time is pretty much impossible to verify. And what is known in the trade as The Vintage Excuse—when a person tries to justify their ratty old stole by saying that it's vintage and therefore the animal was, um, dead already, as opposed to non-vintage furs, which are apparently still alive—is untenable simply because the sale of any fur, vintage or not, promotes the look and feeds the industry. This basically means gullible clothing retailers and fashion fuzz-brains will see you wearing it, potentially think that it is now acceptable, and the trend will reemerge. This goes a million times more so for celebrities, who might think that they're betraying a vaguely dangerous and impressively maverick air by throwing normal considerations to the wind and going out to the Ivy in their new chinchilla coat, when actually all they're doing is proving a long-held theory that anyone who wants to be a celebrity in the first place, who finds that their existence is vindicated only by being photographed, is quite likely to be emotionally, mentally, and intellectually subnormal.

Granted, it is hard to condemn fur and still wear leather. But leather is much harder to live without, and a truly decent alternative that does not have some gratingly pun-tastic name has yet to be invented. Fur, however, is pretty darn easy to do without. Some of us have got by for several decades without wearing any and have yet to suffer hypothermia or feelings of fashion ignominy. Fur supporters like to claim that they "have" to wear fur because it just keeps them so darn cozy. Americans, who are more pro-fur than the Brits, though the latter are certainly catching up, are particularly fond of this justification and yes, absolutely, parts of the United States can be very cold indeed, come winter. But last I heard, New York, for example, does have access to this newfangled invention called "central heating." Fair enough, it does exist only inside, but seeing as the only New Yorkers who spend more than 10 percent of their day outside an office, apartment, coffee shop, or taxi are homeless people, and this is rarely the demographic arguing the case for their Fendi arctic fox stole, it's a tough argument to maintain.

Aside from showing off an apparently rebellious air, one that refuses to bow to sandal-wearing do-gooders banging on about the rights of animals, the other appeal of pelts for fur lovers is that they show off wealth. Second only to jewelry (see **Jewelry, and when fashion just gets obnoxious**), nothing shows off superfluous expenditure better than a big ol' fur, which might explain the remarkable number of crossovers between the jewelry and fur customer bases. Just a fur trim can add hundreds, even thousands to an outfit, and all for the sake of having slightly warmer wrists.

As for arguments that wearing fur is "natural," as proven by the fact that our forebears wore it when they went out hunting woolly mammoths, two replies come to mind: First, this harks back to a time when the term "central heating" referred to two sticks rubbing up against each other in the middle of a cave, and the glaciers were only just beginning to melt, whereas now we have managed to globally heat up this planet so effectively it's a wonder we need coats at all, let alone fur ones. And second, that scary baddies in children's stories almost invariably wear fur, epitomized, of course, by Cruella De Vil, proves that it is instinctive in human nature to equate fur-wearing with evil. And if the fur coat is trimmed with little heads and paws, presumably to keep the wearer company when all sentient human beings have moved away from her in disgust, you can pretty much assume you're dealing with a full-on loon.

Everyone knows about how Naomi Campbell and Cindy Crawford vowed that they would "rather go naked than wear fur" when they posed for a campaign for PETA, only to turn around a few years later and discover that, actually, the latter option wasn't looking too bad these days. Less well known is how these splendid gals justified this impressive turnaround to their rapt followers and, one suspects, themselves.

Crawford, for one, dismissed the public criticism via her publicist, saying that she had never really supported PETA's stand against fur but was instead being "really nice" to the organization when she posed for its campaign in the '90s. Campbell, meanwhile, carried on regardless and is now more commonly seen in court, up on charges for her after-hours hobby of slugging her personal assistants with her bejeweled BlackBerry.

Now I ask you, do you really want to show the world you share the same aesthetic tastes with two such dames? And that's really the main problem with fur: never mind the anal probes, forget about the flashiness, perhaps it's enough that you would be wearing something favored by possibly the most brayingly daft and numbingly stupid people in town. Not a good look, darling.

G-strings, and the female lie

Now, there ain't nothing like a bit of VPL (visible panty line) to make one's backside look three times its normal size, and for this reason women give prostrated thanks for the G-string (though hopefully not while they're wearing one—that would be just disgusting). Anything silk, some light cottons, and the occasional pair of trousers would otherwise be rendered all but unwearable were it not for that bit of anal dental floss. One can't help but think that if these particular clothes were properly made, i.e., had decent linings and so on, then this wouldn't even be an issue, but that, we'll just have to accept, is by the by.

Anyway, somewhere along the line it was decreed that men find this sexy, that looking at a woman with a bit of cotton thread stuck up her bum was the apogee of eroticism. And once Britney Spears was photographed bending over, mid–car clamber, with her G-string hiked above her jeans waistband, well, the nation's women, possibly under mass hypnosis, instantly perceived this as simply the chicest look in town. My gosh, the clever thinking behind it! To show one's G-string proves, first, you are wearing one and, second, that it is now shoved so far up inside, you could probably give yourself a colonoscopy while ordering another mojito at the Soho Lounge. Yes, it was the age of multitasking.

This also cements the lie that women just love to wear strings all the time, denim not generally being a risk for VPL, because secretly, you know, we all just want to dress like bargain basement porn stars. G-strings became yet another example of women wearing something uncomfortable but that they imagined men would find sexy. Men, meanwhile, shruggingly accepted that it must somehow be in women's biological makeup to do this, because *they* sure as hell wouldn't want to walk around all day with a bit of cotton stuck up their arse. Unless they are Peter Stringfellow, of course, a man with a name of nigh-on Dickensian aptness.

It is not a sexy look and it is definitely not a daily one—it's an occasional necessity to be endured, like a padded bra or control-top knickers. And as for G-string bikinis, well, all that needs to be said is, enjoy getting sandy hemorrhoids.

Boyshorts, on the other hand, are sexy and most definitely can be a daily look. They're cute, they're comfy, and, unlike strings, they don't slice into that bulgy bit around your hips, creating not so much a muffin-top effect as a bit of a Michelin Man look. And—strike up the triumphal trumpets—they are sometimes as effective as strings at avoiding VPL but—cue deflationary music—only sometimes. They are also, on a vaguely less sexy note, simply marvelous for communal dressing room moments when you haven't had a bikini wax since, oh, June. Silk, satin, and lace ones are the best to get, for both aesthetic and non-VPL reasons, and for the love of heaven make sure they sit low around your hips. If they don't, you, bless you, have made the error of buying granny pants. High-rise underwear are fine, just a bit dull, and provide neither the bikini-line coverage nor the fantasies about being a 1950s pinup that you get from boyshorts. Admittedly, boyshorts do have an unfortunate gay pedo name, but it's really the man who just loves a bit of G-string that you should worry about, the one who gets off on seeing a lady give herself a cotton enema.

Get: fashion that girls do and boys don't

As anyone who ever watched an episode of *Men Behaving Badly* or perhaps an old Meg Ryan film knows, it is coma-inducingly dull to hash up old gender stereotypes of the "Gosh, aren't men crap/women brilliant/men sensible/women mad" variety. But it seems unlikely that my membership in the gender equality movement will be revoked for stating that sometimes women wear clothes that men just don't get.

Probably the prime example of this is patterns. You see a patterned dress and think, Golly, isn't that summer dress with an old Liberty's print rather fabulously kitsch, with its connotations of England of yore? He thinks, How about that? I never noticed how much she resembles my grandmother's sofa. Ditto with wedges: you're thinking, Kinda cool in a '50s pinup kinda way; he's thinking, Hmmm, orthopedic shoes, just like Old Mother Hubbard probably wore. Prom skirts—How fun, and they make my legs look thin, versus Why is she dressed like the mother in *Back to the Future*? And so the list goes on: tunic dresses, empire lines, cocoon and egg shapes, anything with superfluous buckles and bows, handbags the size of TV sets.

And a response along the lines of "So the hell what?" really does come to mind. First, the idea of buying only clothes that make you look thinner, taller, bustier, or a little like Jennifer

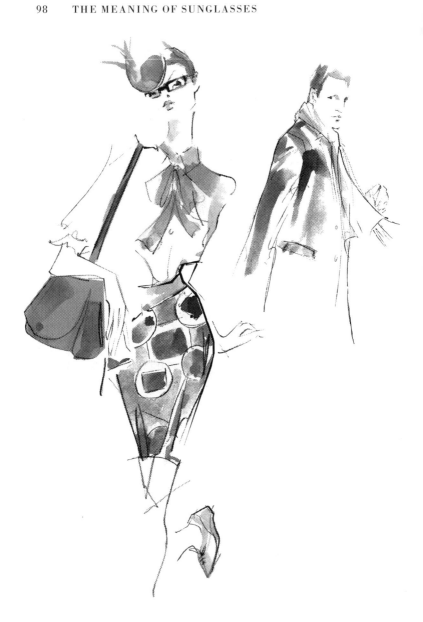

Aniston (pre–pity era) evokes an existence so joyless it makes knowing what a glycemic load is sound like quite a reasonable use of one's brain cells. It's your money. If you only see the point in clothes that garner you appraising looks from slobs on the bus, then fine, off you go and buy yourself yet more mainstream sexy-but-dull jeans, tops, and heels.

If, however, your self-esteem is not predicated on the male gaze, then wear your patterned skirt, pussy-bowed blouse, and your new wedges and enjoy working that (admittedly, a bit too literal) retro secretary look you got going down. Fashion should be about self-expression, and if your self has a little more going for it than worrying about what pleases either of the two pillars of fashion dictatorship—men's mags (tight, short, available) or TV-style makeover shows (fluted sleeves, bias cuts, unthreatening)—then flaunt it to the world, and if they don't like it, that's just too damn bad. Fashion should be something that gives you pleasure; it should not be a logic puzzle to master every morning: "Okay, as I've got short arms I should wear mid-length sleeves, and, with my legs, I need a knee-length skirt."

Moreover, sometimes it's fun just to get on with a fashion trend and to communicate through secret sartorial symbols to other members of our own gender that we, too, read that article in *Glamour* saying we should all try ankle boots with cashmere tights this month. And shouldn't we applaud this? Is it not heartening to realize that sisters are, indeed, doing it for themselves? The rise of labels like the wonky-but-wonderful Marni and frumpy-but-fabulous Prada just proves how deeply this shift has occurred in fashion and in women's approach to fashion in general. Here are two fashion labels that require one to put on one's fashion goggles (aka to have read a fashion magazine) in order to realize you're looking at fashion at all instead of, say, some plain sweaters or baggy tunic dresses. But women love them. And that is why it's called womenswear: it's for the women who wear it. Otherwise it would be called maleonlookerswear, and that's just clunky. This is not to say that one should ignore male opinion entirely. On the contrary, men can be extraordinarily useful simply as a leveler, should you get sartorially carried away. With the noble exceptions of Zandra Rhodes and Italian *Vogue* fashion editor Anna Piaggi, few women really want to wear something that could cause years of trauma to passing children. But this does not mean that one should quash one's own personal taste. Without wishing to drop an "actually-Pamela-Anderson's-aren't-real"–sized bombshell on any male readers, not everything women do is for men. Anyway, it's not as if women sit around wondering why men make themselves deliberately fat and smelly by sitting around all weekend in darkened rooms watching *Match of the Day* like inert bullfrogs. And so, male readers, now another phrase is coming to mind. Wait a minute . . . here it comes . . . oh yes: "Deal."

Glasses, and why men will still make passes

There may be less of a stigma about astigmatism these days, but women still seem to fear wearing glasses more than men. Odd, really, considering how fond many of them are of slipping on sunglasses—but then, of course, sunglasses suggest glamour, whereas the untinted ones are redolent of Milhouse tendencies (Milhouse, Bart Simpson's best friend, that is, not his namesake, Richard Milhous Nixon, although the latter isn't really an icon of feminine appeal either—or of good spectacle choices).

The idea that men shy away from women in glasses seems a little unfair to their gender, inferior though they may be. Perhaps more to the point, if glasses are sartorial shorthand for smarts, one has to wonder what fearing to wear them says about a woman. Maybe some men do run in disgust from a nearsighted lady, but unless your goal in life is to become a Playboy bunny, it's unlikely this will ultimately prove too much of a hurdle in your search for love and companionship. And so we have yet another instance of men being underestimated by the rest of the planet and women's insecurities making them behave like loons. But don't feel too guilty: even Marilyn Monroe did it in *How to Marry a Millionaire*—the iconic movie for all squinting ladies—bumping along aimlessly through life, squired by undeserving shallow men, until she finally put on her fabulous glasses, looked totally brilliant, and shacked up with a bankrupt spy. It's astonishing that this universal lesson has yet to sink in with the rest of the world.

In any event, there is something rather sexy about glasses. They become another, particularly intimate, thing to remove at carefully chosen moments. And because they so affect your appearance, to show how you look without them reveals a hidden layer, a secret self, even. So don't be so keen to pop in the contact lenses: why not keep something of your naked appearance hidden for the special few?

Glasses can so redefine your face that they work almost like makeup. And like makeup, they need to be updated as your face shape changes. Don't get stuck in a rut, whether it be an overreliance on gold eye shadow or oval frames.

And also as with makeup, the best thing to do is to keep it subtle, so no glasses with turned-up corners like those of some coquettish 1950s secretary. These are the desperate pleas of the optically insecure: "Yes, I may need glasses, but look! See how girly and feminine they are? Honestly, I don't read that much!" Similar story for patterned frames ("I'm more wacky than smart, you know") or circular ("Like, I'm all about peace, man, so any comments about my glasses are just displays of your shallowness"). Obviously, if you're lucky enough to wear glasses you should have fun with them. Just don't use them to send out messages that don't need to be said. Honestly, you can rely on your personality to overcome any lingering stereotypes and, anyway, the classy people will be able to see—sniff!—the true person behind them.

Hair accessories: gimmicks for reluctant adults

Definitely one of the cleverer offshoots of accessories madness (see **Accessories: going to hell in a handbag**). Designers wisely prepared the ground for this state of affairs with the ever-rising cost of accessories in general, but designer hair accessories are truly the heroin of the fashion industry, in that they must be the ultimate example of 1,000 percent markups. A lovely young British woman called Katie Hillier can take a lot of credit for this, as she is the woman behind many of the pieces that the king and queen of tempting knickknacks, Marc Jacobs and Luella, have been knocking out for years, particularly their oversized logoed hair baubles. Miu Miu and Prada, similarly, have been making pretty feathered and glittery headbands for some time, convincing women who really should know better to pay triple figures for—and I would like to emphasize this for a second time—a headband. Aside from the fact that you are likely to lose your designer hair accessory after one wear, they are not quite as daft as you think; a pretty hair accessory distracts from a bad-hair cut/day/life and a sparkly hair band will do more than a gallon of Touche Eclat to make you look a bit perkier and party-tastic. Feathered headbands, particularly ones that match the color of your hair, are possibly the easiest way to add some pleasing glamour to an outfit that even you are sick of seeing yourself wearing. Frankly, it's a lot easier to stick a headband in your hair than to figure out how the hell one is supposed to put on liquid eyeliner without resembling Marilyn Manson.

But it's the word "headband" that causes a lot of women in this country to quail, and understandably so. One must always be on one's guard against the sneaking dominance of preppiness, and headbands, sadly, are very much the sartorial symbol of this demographic. A pity, really, because the truth is, most women look better with their hair neatly tucked back. That so many of them often wear their sunglasses pushed up on their head proves that they know this, and it is a real shame that they are forced to make do with this pathetic compromise just because they fear the stigma of the headband. (And any of you ladies out there weakly protesting that you only do this sunglasses trick for "convenience' " sake, ask yourselves, how often do you see a man wearing his shades on his head?) Shake off the shackles of fear, you sad, repressed ladies, and just get yourself a pretty headband, jeweled, sequined, feathered, or a simple black one. Never get a plastic or wooden one as it will squeeze your head like some medieval torture instrument. Velvet-coated bands are the most comfortable; thin ones are good for a pretty, vaguely French style, and wide ones are there for when you're wanting to work a bit of a '60s look. The difficulty with hair accessories in general is that they can easily shade into the pedo chic territory, but this, too, is unfair. Quite why only children are allowed to sport things to keep their hair tidy when it is unquestionably adults who reap the harsher criticism for going around with a scruffy bird's-nest-ian mop makes little sense. Not everyone has the time, money, or patience for a weekly $200 blow-dry, you know. Admittedly, the hair accessories industry has not helped itself on this score by decking the majority of hair baubles and whatnots with multi-colored charms and Hello Kitty characters, but one must fight this vicious circle, if only for the sake of easy, tidy hair. In terms of hair baubles—hair bands with little knickknacks attached—simpler is best, and monochrome is best of all. Yes, baubles are more fun than a plain hairband, but restrain yourself and step away from the pink hearts; you will only compound skeptics' prejudices against hairbands and simultaneously make yourself look like a complete twit. So reach instead for oversized black or white balls, tortoiseshell cubes, or something similar and mini-malist (well, as minimalist as you can get with a hair bauble).

Scrunchies manage to beat even the headband in terms of unfortunate image association. Forever associated with '80s aer-obics classes and car pool mothers, the scrunchie has defied the skills of even the most determined fashion stylist to resurrect this accessory, even on an ironic level, and it's really not worth both-ering. Unlike the beleaguered headband, a scrunchie improves no one's look—it's sloppy, it's clunky, and it doesn't even hold your hair in properly. *Quel,* as the French probably don't say, *est le point?*

Haircuts: the meaning beneath the layers

We've all heard, thanks to that universal hairdresser opening spiel, that haircuts are dependent on face shape. But in truth, we all know that the only thing to bear in mind when choosing a haircut is what it says about you.

This is why women get so stressed about their hair. Aside from the general complaints pretty much every woman save Tinsley Mortimer (the goddess of hair) has regarding her hair, it is this tonsorial message that causes the angst. No single garment, nay, not even a word out of your mouth will create as much of an immediate first impression as your haircut. But, you know, no pressure.

The youthful pixie cut is one such example. Here is a haircut that says "I am young and I have heard the word 'gamine' and I like it. I am ethereal and above material concerns like buying conditioner. But such spiritualism in no way conflicts with my desire to show off what I have been told are my very good cheekbones." For the older woman, this cut tends to be indicative of an exchange of vanity for deeper, more cerebral concerns, as though you are too busy campaigning for Sudanese refugees or memorizing Shakespearean soliloquies to brush your hair in the mornings (ref: Judi Dench). But it can look a bit like you just can't be bothered anymore.

The bob is an interesting one, as this sends different messages depending on what side of the social spectrum you're coming from. Because long hair is still synonymous with youth, it's either the compromising style of a woman who reckons that her long feminine locks, on which she relied for the first twenty-nine years of her life, just aren't suitable anymore, but she's not in any way ready for the middle-aged crop (see above)—grown-up but still pretty, in other words, while wisely ducking the yummy mummy cliché of opting for long hair to swing about one's shoulders in front of the school gates. Or it's the aspiration to thinking-girl status for a pop star or socialite, though it says something about both of these demographics that lopping off three inches of hair is considered proof of one's maverick intelligence. The bob is a fairly limiting hairstyle, and it requires the same amount of confidence as the pixie cut, because you are going to be stuck looking at the same reflection in the mirror for the next six months. For this reason, it is also very popular with women who are or just wish to look very professional and busy, because there is absolutely nothing that needs to or can be done with it. Anna Wintour is the icon; Betty Boop is the occasional outcome.

The gateway to the bob, bangs, work in a similar manner but with whole new levels of semiotics and suggestion. Somehow, this Goody Two-shoes style has recently acquired an edgy kind of image. Once it brought to mind images of overgrown children's TV presenters; now it is more redolent of the slightly cooler Karen from the Yeah Yeah Yeahs. This is mainly because it works in the same way as the pixie cut and bob, in that it is suggestive of confidence in one's appearance because, ultimately, once you have a fringe, there is not much more you can do to your hair, as it's just going to sit there like a pudding. Of course, the real boon of bangs, which probably explains more fully their sudden popularity, is that they are painless Botox, a forehead wrinkle cover-up. In this sense, it is basically the posh version of what was once known as, to use the probably not politically correct term, a white trash face-lift, which involved pulling back one's hair into a ponytail so tight your face looked like Han Solo's at the beginning of *Return of the Jedi* as he strained to get out of his wall tomb.

Because bangs themselves have become so popular, even the type of fringe you have has become fraught with meaning: do you go for the "I'm a bit quirky and did I mention I live in a, like, totally gritty warehouse," slightly-too-short, wonky style? Or perhaps the mainstream-pop-star diagonal long cut, perfect for looking up to the right and batting your M.A.C.-coated eyelashes? Or maybe the preppishly long and thick version—again, very useful for eyelash battage? Know thyself, choose thy bangs, as Yoda might well have said, should he have pondered the matter. The best kind is the long and thick version, but this does depend on your having thick hair to begin with; otherwise you will use up half the hair that should be around your skull to sit atop your forehead, which not only isn't very attractive but also looks silly and creates the female equivalent of the male comb-over.

Layering is the bootcut jean of the tonsorial world, with its mainstream feminine appeal and obvious benefits (it vaguely makes your hair look thicker), but the equally pressing disadvantages (you now have completely uneven hair that will look like a total bird's nest as soon as you try to grow it out). Yet like the bootcut, such detractions have wielded notably little sway, and layers continue to be the most popular style for women, possibly due to too many seminal years of watching Farrah Fawcett followed by her '80s aspirants flick their short and long bits around with such fabulous insouciance.

And then there's the most popular hairstyle of all: the shoulder-length opt-out. This is the female hair equivalent of the commitment-phobic boy: you know you're getting on a bit, you know you really should let go of some of those hang-ups you've had since you were fifteen—but somehow you just can't quite make the leap to having a proper haircut. Too scary, too high maintenance, too expensive, you imagine. In fact, just as lurching aimlessly from relationship to relationship is probably more expensive and exhausting than just settling down, so having to get your shapeless shoulder-length style trimmed every six weeks is far more tedious and less heartwarming than just embracing a proper cut.

But at least women can have a bit of fun with their hair without risking accusations of effeminacy or general pretension. Men undoubtedly have it much worse, mainly because they must work within a smaller framework and thus the slightest alteration has a much greater and potentially more damaging impact. There's the aging-lothario quiff, that of an older gent who walks through life with the optimistic words "silver fox" dancing through his head and is so proud of maintaining his thick locks he quiffs them up to a gravity-defying and -denying degree (ref: Robert Redford, Warren Beatty).

This tendency to be so proud of one's assets that one then flaunts them to an inadvisable degree is a common mistake made by both men and women, in hair and nonhair matters. With women, it tends to be in regard to thinness or breast size, leading, in the case of the former, either to overly cinched dresses, too-high miniskirts, or pedophile chic. ("I'm so little I can still fit into Gap Kids, giggle giggle." The correct answer to this is, "Yeah, you must be really grateful that the childhood obesity problem has helped to widen your wardrobe choices.") In regard to the latter, the obvious result is a cleavage that rivals the Grand Canyon, gloriously on display to potential tourists and hapless onlookers (see **Cleavage, and the plumbing of depths**).

Going back to men's hair, there's the "head 'em off at the first post" style, otherwise known as shaving your head at the initial sign of balding, as if, actually, you always intended to have a naked scalp, so this is really a good thing, and what do you mean you found a bottle of Rogaine in my bathroom? The short back and sides is always safe, if a little retro (fashion-speak for "dull"), and the lightly feathered cut, aka the male Judi Dench, tends to be favored by self-conscious men's magazine editors—who think such geekiness is a bit, y'know, ironic.

No more need be said in regard to the comb-over ever since the truly seminal Oprah Winfrey show in which she cut off men's comb-overs. Oprah, not even that school you set up in Africa has demonstrated more succinctly why you were put on this planet.

Name me a single time when long hair has improved a man's looks and I will personally come round to your house and tap dance naked on your coffee table. The nadir is the long but balding cut, creating a wilting-crop-circle effect on a gentleman's head. It is so easy to see the train of thought here: "I'll compensate for the lack of hair upon my head by growing it to hang around my jowls." But as is always the case with fashion, when the intention is obvious, the effect is simply unacceptable. (See **Animal print: when women roar.** Or for that matter, Michael Bolton.)

Hair extensions, and when you realize you no longer understand the young

Every generation must have its defining beauty treatment, one that is as misguided as it is painful. In the '70s it was the sun bed, in the '80s it was the oversized perm. For a while, it looked like the early-twenty-first century's contribution to the cosmetic historic annals would be the glycolic acid peel, a treatment that looked as horrid as you'd expect from something with the word "acid" in it. But hair extensions have unquestionably stolen this tarnished crown, making them the foot binding of the modern Western world.

Long, thick hair is still equated with youthful beauty. But here we have yet another example of an idea taken far beyond the realms of pleasing aesthetics. Just as the predominance of underweight teenage models on the catwalks shows the nasty side of thin, so the sight of nineteen-year-olds gluing bits of Russian peasants' hair onto their scalps and then boredly picking dried bits of glue suggests that luxuriant locks aren't necessarily a gateway to sexiness.

It's hard to pinpoint when hair extensions first began their determined prowl, but by 2002 it was the rare manufactured female pop star who didn't have some fake hair glued to her head. As a procedure, it was painstaking and painful; as a look, it was obvious and cheap. Glossy celebrity magazines were packed full of pictures of homogeneous women strolling through the streets of central LA and New York with their fake nails, fake tans, and, now, fake hair—great tails of the stuff sitting chunkily within their own genuine material. The benefit to this was, one could say in all honesty that our celebrities were fake from top to toe without any fear of libel, seeing as the growing popularity of strappy sandals also prompted a rise in fake toenails, allowing one to hide one's scabby yellow versions beneath rather spooky plastic white ones. The downside was that, where the C-list lady celebs go, the teenage masses must follow. And so it was that, while sifting through the harmless dangling earrings and "gold-style" necklaces one finds in Claire's Accessories and similar emporiums, one would find one's wrist being attacked by what appeared to be a toothless honey-blond ferret, only to realize that it was a horrid nylon hair extension.

Some were bound in the hair with ties, some still went down the glue route (much more fun to pick at); neither looked the least bit natural. Most tended to be fake, real hair being (a) a little expensive and (b) slightly nauseating. Natural-looking hair was a bit passé anyway. Multicolored stripes were suddenly the sign of a classy, high-maintenance lifestyle. Both nylon extensions and heavy blond highlights gave women's hair across the land the look of a tiger's hide. Hairdressers welcomed this expensive trend by making noises about how it added "movement" and "depth" and other words these professionals are able to spout with commendably sober faces. The pop group McFly sang longingly about "The Girl with Five Colors in Her Hair," and apparently that was a good thing, rather than the clash between a heavy hand and a home dyeing kit. Actually, what it showed was that women love to have a new and expensive beauty treatment, quality of the results be damned, whether it be striping their hair or having cucumber water rubbed into their skin beneath the sound of wind chimes (see **Beauty treatments, and the etiquette thereof**). It's a combination of the self-indulgence and self-reassurance deriving from the conviction that they are fighting the onslaught of aging and even better maintaining themselves. Never mind that hair extensions frizz up in the rain, making them resemble Charles III at his bewigged finest—they are looking after themselves as a modern lady should.

But with the exception of Hugh Hefner, men aren't usually keen on fakeness in women. It is a rare male who dreams of finding his ideal woman and running his fingers through her nylon locks. And if you've ever seen a young man's facial expression when he realizes that what seemed at first so fulsome and curvy was, in fact, just sponge and padding and is now lying on the bedroom floor, you can just about get the idea of his reaction when he spots tails of his beloved's tonsorial beauteousness lying around the bathroom sink in a gluey mess. Obviously, male queasiness is no reason not to do something. But as it certainly cannot give one any personal pleasure, surely there is little other reason to stick bits of hair onto one's scalp. Thus, we have yet another example of Women Doing Something They Think Men Will Like But Which Actually Makes Them Look Like Complete Freaks.

Even more ridiculous is the fact that when you get your hair extensions changed, which you have to do regularly, you need to cut out the bits of your hair to which they are bound, thus making your naturally thin hair even thinner.

Certainly, clip-on fake ponytails are rather jolly for special occasions.

But just as it's far more satisfying to eat a little bit of natural butter than to load up on the synthetic fake stuff, so it is wiser to accept the depleted locks God gave you—jazzing them up a bit with some nice hair accessories—than to mess about with bits of scraggly nylon.

Haute couture: taking self-indulgence to a whole new level

Everything about the haute couture industry is self-indulgent, from the women spending $100,000 and seventy hours being measured for a made-to-measure dress decked with gold tassels and beading to the designers staging huge shows in which models visibly wilt under the weight of their Elizabethan ball gowns, crusader helmets, and medieval-weaponry-influenced accessories, all in the name of conveying the designer's self-professed fascination with "strong women" (here's a hint, designer friend o mine: if you're so interested in strong women, why not just get some models who actually weigh more than one hundred pounds?) to the journalists making the biannual schlep to the shows in Paris to write about clothes that, unless they work for *Majesty* magazine, not a single one of their readers will ever wear to the celebrities shipped in to make their requisite front-row appearance all in the name of getting a bit more attention for themselves and the designer without even the mitigating possibility that they are likely to wear these clothes to anywhere other than the Oscars.

Most people's idea of a fashion show is based on the couture model instead of the more proletariat prêt-à-porter. Couture is the perfume oil to prêt-à-porter's eau de parfum: a more concentrated version and, as such, with a decidedly stronger, occasionally overpowering effect. Certainly prêt-à-porter has its moments, but fashion's long-maintained reputation for theatrical silliness would be seriously dented if people knew that the majority of the ready-to-wear shows involved models wearing plain trousers and floaty dresses and, in short, looking like normal women—conspicuously well dressed women, admittedly—on their way to meet friends for lunch. So thank heavens for the pyrotechnics of couture to keep the fires of the old stereotypes burning brightly.

Just as every fashion journalist has to write, at least twice a year, a halfhearted article weakly waving the flag for their national fashion industry—despite the fact that even the fashion designers seem to have realized this is a lost cause, judging from the way they all flee their respective cities at the first sniff of success and head to Paris—so every fashion journalist in the world needs to write a biannual article justifying the ongoing couture industry. It's the tax you pay for having found a way to make a career out of talking about dresses and shopping.

There's no real justification for couture—of course there isn't. Maybe back in Marie Antoinette's day when there was nothing to do but lie around all afternoon eating pastry and taxing peasants, idling away hours being fitted for one bed jacket and then spending more on a dress than most people earned in a lifetime made just the most marvelous sense. Now that we live in an H&M, Zara world, such a concept holds somewhat less appeal.

The fact that the few people left on this planet who do have the time, money, and capacity for this kind of sheer self-indulgence are such an undeniably unappealing bunch has not helped couture's image. Minor European royals, overfed bankers' wives, Ivana Trump—the word "aspirational" does not come to mind here.

The most commonly used justifications for couture wheeled out by the desperate fashion hack are that it provides a "springboard" for the designer's creativity; that designers can practice the more extreme variations of their styles for next season in the welcoming hothouse of the couture world; and that it allows them to "experiment" more. Aside from conjuring up the appealing image of designers as mad scientists mixing crazy potions while wearing neat white lab coats (very Maison Martin Margiela, incidentally—a label in which the publicists actually do wear lab coats, but that's a whole other bag of potatoes), this theory just does not wash. Of course designers need to experiment and, yes, they might need to work through various versions of a style before they arrive at the watered-down, wearable conclusion. But why does a whole industry need to be based on what are essentially designers' first drafts?

The other argument is that couture is not fashion—it's art. The ol' "Is fashion art?" article is even more boring and tired than the "What is the point of couture?" one. Fashion has to be wearable, otherwise it is not clothes, and it may as well be a medieval artifact in the Natural History Museum. Certainly the work that goes into couture clothes is impressive, judging from statements that buzz around the couture shows like pesky flies, such as "That dress took ninety hours for one seamstress to make" and "The beads on that bodice were culled from an endangered oyster." But again, this does not justify an industry. And if it's just art, why is it tied to the commercial structure of fashion seasons? I don't seem to remember hearing that Leonardo da Vinci ever thought, "You know, I'd really fancy knocking out another painting this month, but it's October, and I only produce my wares for the public twice a year in order to fit in with store ordering systems and fashion shoot schedules."

The only justification for couture is that it's fun. Couture is the fashion world writ large, with its silly shows, its pretentious inspirations, and its hilarious price tags. Thus, it demonstrates more clearly than anywhere else that the only point of fashion itself is to have fun. You can try to find as many justifications as you like—it expresses the political situation, perhaps, or maybe it Reflects the Zeitgeist—but ultimately, it's about enjoying clothes, and there really is no other excuse at all for couture than that. You can't even use the vague excuse that you have for prêt-à-porter, which is that people need clothes and therefore it is providing them a service; not even Ivana Trump, I'd wager, would claim that anyone needs a $60,000 bolero jacket. In short, couture is a sharp lesson in the realities of the fashion world and proof of how one just has to lean back and enjoy it. And if that puts a conclusive end to all those articles about whether fashion is art or about the political significance of a long hem, well, I'd say that it provides a darn good service to all mankind.

Heels: the highs, the lows, and when fat is better than thin

Enjoy this sentence while you can, because you're unlikely to hear it in regard to anything else in the fashion world: Fat is sud-

denly better than thin. This, at first, would seem not to make a
jot of sense. The whole theory behind heels—indeed, the only
excuse for them—is that men allegedly find them sexy. Now is
not the time to delve too deeply into why any man would find
a limping woman with overly developed, Barbie doll arches
attractive (or perhaps we have just answered the question), but
rather let us just accept that, if this is the case, then a thin, delicate heel is definitely sexier than a clunking great tubster.

A spindly spike perpetuates the illusion that a woman is a
Tinker Bell–like creature who can float through the air, her feet
supported only by toothpicks, such is her lightness. This is a
delicate flower, it says, who never sweats,
belches, or bleeds. A chunky heel, however, suggests that the woman might
actually have some disgusting body
weight that needs a bit of support.

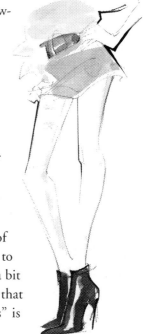

The brilliant thing about the sudden and surprising emergence of the
thick heel—aside from the fact that,
after 2,000 years, shoemakers seem to
have come to grips with the idea of
weight distribution—is that it doesn't
look like you're trying so hard to be
sexy, and this, in itself, is sexier.

Fashion magazines are very fond of
using the word "insouciance" in regard to
this look, possibly because it sounds a bit
French and it's quite fun to show off that
you know how to spell it. "Effortless" is

another popular one, even if the word does ring false when talking about a $1,200 Miu Miu boot and an $1,800 Marni sack dress.

The only exception to this thin is bad, fat is good rule is to use its Latin name, the Sparklius Girlsnightoutus, otherwise known as the strappy sandal, which leaves the foot near naked with only a couple of strands of rhinestone or, for the classier sorts, leather ribbon ties, to hold it in place. The strappy sandal is such a determined return to the obvious that to bother with all this faux frumpier-is-actually-sexier-than-sex nonsense would be just as pointless as eating a salad mid–chocolate pig-out.

Another and perhaps less psychologically complex reason for the emergence of fat heels—and cone heels, while we're here, which are one step further down on the unsexy-heel spectrum and, thus, a great favorite of unsexy-womenswear designers like Marc Jacobs and Marni—is that they serve the same purpose as wedges and platforms in drawing attention to the shoe. Women have long been a little weird about shoes, and the Freudian theories behind this are too boring and too obvious to elaborate. (Oh, okay, fine. Obviously, it's all about sex with all that insertion of the foot and penetration of the shoe, or whatever. God forbid women should do anything that is not somehow connected to sexual desire for a man, as opposed to, say, just being materialistic and fancying a pair of shoes.) But this interest in showing off the shoe itself as opposed to one's own appearance has emerged with the rise in accessory mania (see **Accessories: going to hell in a handbag**). Well, if you're going to spend $400 on a pair of Burberry ankle boots, you might as well have people notice them.

The issue of heel width and height is a fraught one indeed.

The famous, nigh-on historical, really, "fuck-me shoes" standoff between Germaine Greer and Suzanne Moore clarified two issues: One, perhaps the feminist movement wasn't working out too well if one of its leading lights was going around town like some ascetic priest accusing her followers of slatternly behavior. And two, that after all these years, the feminist debate about fashion—conforming to a misogynistic interpretation of beauty versus women enjoying themselves—still hadn't been resolved. In fact, Germaine rather missed the point here, because stilettos don't suggest that a woman is betraying her feminist roots by trying to look like a slut, they suggest that she is totally daft and has absolutely no understanding of the concept of weight distribution, and this, I'd have thought, is actually a worse betrayal of the equality dream.

It is the oddest concept, and it would have been interesting to see how it was first pitched: "Hey, guys! Let's make shoes that force women to walk on their tippy-toes all day! Shoes that require them to take a taxi to travel to the end of the road!" "Amazing! Crank up the machines!"

And yet, here we are, hundreds of millions of women daily hoisting themselves up onto the balls of their feet in the name of fashion, spending hundreds and hundreds, and in some cases thousands, of dollars on shoes that they literally cannot walk in. "Wow, loving your shoes!" "Yeah, they're great. Can't really walk in them, of course, but they look fabulous." Really, it's like saying, "Yes, I love my new car. Of course, the engine is totally buggered, but I love to just sit in it, not going anywhere." Stilettos make women

  (a) grumpy,
  (b) lazy (due entirely to immobility), and
  (c) pathetically slow.

All, one would have thought, quite unattractive qualities. And yet, and yet, the myth persists that stilettos are sexy.

One theory is that they force the woman's foot into the shape it makes when having a Meg Ryan moment and thus give off the image that she is sexually available. However, seeing as a woman mid-orgasm tends to be, shall we say, already taken and therefore the very opposite of available, one can only assume that "sexually available" really means the woman puts out. Which is nice. Others argue that the appeal of the high heel lies in the way it emphasizes a woman's curvy—fertile—shape. Kinda sweet, isn't it, to think that after all these years of evolution, all a man really wants to see is that his woman is fertile, even if he doesn't actually—oh God, no, don't even raise the specter of the possibility—want to have a child with her. As I said, sweet. But perhaps women should ask themselves if they really want to walk around town looking like Nubian fertility symbols.

This is not to deny that high heels can be fun. Yes, they're glamorous and, yes, they're quite fun to dance in (for a few minutes, after which they become excruciating), as you can look down at your feet and pretend that you're Ginger Rogers. But accept that there is quite a disadvantage to this heels nonsense—namely, you can't walk in them—and that perhaps the "cons" sometimes cancel out the "pros."

The idea that stilettos are somehow "dressier" and that flats are too "casual" for a party just doesn't wash. There are so many pretty, dainty flats out there and so very many hideous, clunky, square-toed heels. Moreover, if you wear flats to a party, you'll dash about all night like a veritable social dynamo, giggling ever so gaily, living it up on the dance floor, and leaving bedazzled men in your wake. Wear stilettos and you'll spend the evening slumped uncomfortably in the corner or searching for a chair before you finally give it up, take off your shoes, and show the world your cracked heels and hammertoes.

As for the kitten heel, really, the only thing to say here is that one should never trust anything with such a repulsively stupid name. What on earth could a squashed little heel have to do with the feline family?

The problem with the kitten heel is that, as happens with most compromises, you get the worst of both worlds. You have to grip the wretched things with your toes just to get them to stay on your feet, making your calves swell up like waterlogged balloons. And this, as all ladies know, is always a great look. If you really are dead set on wearing a heel, get either a smallish (but not kitten) slender one or a high one of a good four or five inches that is satisfyingly chunky.

But really, to see the cold facts about heels, just wait until the end of a party and watch the women leave. While those in flats glide easily out the door and dash lightly down the road to grab the last bus home, those in heels can barely hobble. Their bodies limp slowly down the road, knees jutting forward, back hunching downward, like *Homo sapiens* emerging from the swamps. Thus, flatswearers are, on all levels, more highly evolved. So there.

Hems: the highs and lows (part 2)

Even though most discussions regarding hems tend to focus on the issue of short versus long, this, actually, is the easiest topic on the table. Here, the only word you need to bear in mind is "balance." If you're flashing a lot of leg, keep your top half reasonably covered, unless you particularly want to resemble a Big Brother reject. Floaty tops, sloppy V-neck sweaters, and pretty blouses all work well with miniskirts, as do straight jackets and blazers. If the idea of wearing something voluminous sparks worries that people will assume you are Jabba the Hutt beneath the layers, take succor from the fact that your non-Jabba-esque legs will be on view, so people will probably have a good idea of your actual general shape. This also stops the miniskirt from looking too self-consciously sexy and keeps it in its rightful place of being something to have fun in that makes you feel good and not on general display. Long skirts, meanwhile, obviously need to be worn with something a little more form-fitting. Otherwise, you will be occasionally overtaken by the urge to break into "Climb Ev'ry Mountain." Both high and low hems look best with flat shoes, and everything in between generally requires a bit of height adjustment.

But—ah!—what a sign of innocence to see this as the end of the matter. As with jeans (see **Jeans: not as bulletproof as they tell you**), the human species has made the issue of hems into a subject that rivals the Good Friday Agreement in complexities and potential for disaster (probably).

Take tissue hems (please, et cetera, and so forth). These are very popular among the tackier echelons of the mass market because of their cheap-to-make, attention-grabbing appearance. They are also a favored style of self-described molto sexy designers, such as Roberto Cavalli, thanks to their suggestion of untrammeled, almost primal sexuality. They give you the look of having just emerged from the jungle, leaving behind the exhausted body of a man you've just savaged (and who presumably ripped your hem with mid-coital excitement).

In truth, they just make most women look like they are playing Titania in a community theater production of *A Midsummer Night's Dream.* There is something so grating in the faux spontaneity of the tissue hem, as though its jaggedness were the result of some recent wild ambush, as opposed to some poor guy in a factory carefully measuring and cutting triangular shapes in the fabric just so. And because of the awkward interchanging length issue—okay, it's a long dress, oops, no, it's a short one, oh no, wait, it's long again—it is very difficult to judge what kind of shoes to wear and whether it's acceptable to wear tights with it (not that I'm encouraging the adoption of this look, but, should you insist, the correct answers are, respectively, strappy sandals and no, which is God's way of telling you that the only time tissue hems are just about acceptable is on beach holidays).

If you are the kind of person, though, who insists on having a bit of fun with their hem, well, first, you might want to get out more. If that doesn't quench the desire, the fishtail hem—when a dress gets deliberately longer at the back—is a far better choice than the tissue. It is just that little bit more subtle and, compared to the shrill silliness of its tissue colleague, it looks quietly glamorous. A bit bridal, perhaps, and for that reason it is best to get one that doesn't quite touch the ground but rather ends midway down your calf, with the front of the dress ending at your knees. This length also serves to head off the risk of an aquatic appearance, which the dress's name kindly warns one about but is often overlooked by ladies, judging by the number of aquamarine or silver full-length fishtail dresses that can be spotted at any wedding party.

The fishtail also makes a nice change from the all-too-numerous dresses and skirts out there that always are too short at the back because of manufacturers' forgetting that women occasionally have this odd anatomical feature called "a bum" that deigns to take up some of the garment's fabric to cover itself, meaning that short skirts and dresses are almost always just that little bit too skimpy at the back. The fishtail hem allows a woman to experience the novel sensation of not spending an evening tugging down the back of her skirt.

The bias cut is also a perfectly pretty style but one that has sadly been condemned to cliché hell. Its wavelike hem led to various theories centering on its potential to "slim the legs," leading to its becoming quite the favorite of women's-magazine fashion shoots and TV makeover harridans. Yet most bias-cut skirts end two or three inches below the knee, i.e., at the widest part of the calf, which pretty much destroys all leg-slimming potential, even if you sewed a whole darn tsunami of waves into the hem.

Jacobs, Marc: genius or what?

Genius, actually, since you ask, and not just because he makes such nice things that—shock, gasp—actually last forever. Rather, it's how he has made a breathtakingly lucrative career for himself by mining an image for his label that is so utterly at odds with what he produces.

There are many other indicators of his brilliance—not least the way he made fashion cool again—but number one has to be how he convinced the world that his label conveyed an image of downtown, cool creative chic, of young film directors having black coffee on the Lower East Side as opposed to ritzied-up wives of bankers meeting for lunch at Barneys on Madison Avenue. Quite how $2,500 bags with giant gold chains and $6,000 floor-length dresses fit in with this idea of ascetic garret living is anyone's guess, but nonetheless Jacobs managed to convince the world. And how did he do this? By palling around with Sofia Coppola (a Hollywood progeny who is seen as trendy, primarily because she doesn't wear makeup and rarely smiles) and having Jürgen Teller (a hugely successful photographer, who has a vaguely gritty reputation thanks to his askew and frequently overbleached pictures) shoot his advertising campaign. Wow, keep it real, Marc. Make fun of the artifice and importance of brand image all you like, but at least those of, for example, Dolce & Gabbana and Valentino (respectively, scary-rich Italian ladies and scary-rich ladies in general) bear a modicum of truth in relation to their customer base. Marc Jacobs's advertised demographic couldn't even afford to buy one of his key chains. In fact, many of the same people who buy Valentino buy Marc

Jacobs, it's just that they feel slightly cooler when they buy the latter.

In part, Jacobs's success reflects the general gentrification of New York City. Over the past fifteen years, downtown has become just as chichi as uptown. But the fact remains, Jacobs's image is based on an idea of left-field, artsy-slacker cool, not, as would probably be more accurate of both his downtown neighborhood and customer demographic, trust fund kids plowing Daddy's life savings into the ground. Yet to mock is self-defeating, because it is thanks to this truly impressive PR campaign that Jacobs regenerated the fashion world. Sure, fashion was always desirable, but by the early '90s it was all shoulder pads and ladies who lunch—profitable, perhaps, but not exactly cutting edge. Then scrawny, geeky, bespectacled Jacobs came along, put grunge on the catwalk, got photographed hanging out with cool celebrities like Sonic Youth and Evan Dando, made clothes for twenty-somethings as well as the older market, and suddenly fashion became a young person's game. Labels such as Miu Miu, Luella, Stella McCartney, and the rejuvenated Chloé all owe something to Jacobs, because he really did pave a path, generally to the bank accounts of improbably wealthy under-twenty-five-year-olds around the world.

And by making fashion younger, especially through his fantastic diffusion label Marc by Marc Jacobs, he also showed the mass market how to make good clothes for teenagers that were a step above the scratchy cropped tops and saggy denim skirts it had been relying on previously. H&M, in particular, has learned a lot from Jacobs: mainly that the customer does notice little details, such as contrasting piping on the seams of hooded tops or oversized buttons on cardigans, and that for a retailer, cutting sleeves properly so they make your arms look slim—as opposed to letting them bag sloppily under your armpits—could make the difference between breaking even and busting all profit records.

With so many followers, perhaps it is understandable that Jacobs is thinking these days about, on the one hand, the more la-di-da end of the market with his mainline collections and, on the other, the cheap and cheerful end of the spectrum with his diffusion label, knocking out heart-shaped plastic compacts and rubber beach shoes like he'd never heard the words "image control," thus increasingly shucking any pretensions to downtown hipster status. He is now creative director of Louis Vuitton, perhaps the most monied and least cool label around, and has said that his dream job is to work at Chanel, the ultimate bastion of the very same ladies who lunch who controlled fashion before his grunged-up emergence. *Plus ça change,* eh? And yet, because he still looks like the school geek and still name-checks Sofia (who has herself moved on from slacker-tastic *Lost in Translation* to, rather aptly, *Marie Antoinette*), he is still seen as the acceptably cool face of fashion. But then image, you know, is everything.

Jeans: not as bulletproof as they tell you

Ah, bless the human species. No sooner does it find something pretty straightforward than it has to fuss with it, divesting it of many of its original charms. (See **Classics with a twist.**)

And so it has been with jeans. We all know the story: once jeans were kind of cool in a James Dean way; then they were the favored uniform of the American tourist, who decided that wearing high-waisted, tapered trousers in bleached denim was a sure way to cut a fine figure. And then in the '90s, a clever little jeans label called Earl moved the waistband slightly lower, put a bit of stretch into the denim, and—wham bam, your receipt's in the bag, ma'am—jeans are suddenly the most flattering thing ever conceived in the history of civilization. New denim labels are launched every day with increasingly self-important names (Citizens of Humanity, True Religion, 7 For All Mankind—I mean, I ask you) and reported in the fashion press with the kind of hushed excitement more suited to breaking news of the Second Coming of Christ. Designer jeans now easily cost over $300, making them more expensive than a lot of designer shoes. Yet their cost has not affected their popularity in the slightest, and, like handbags and cosmetics, they are increasingly one of the financial pillars of many fashion brands.

And so manufacturers, understandably, decided to milk this cash cow for all it was worth, experimenting with every possible style, design, and color variation they could possibly imagine in order to convince customers to buy more, more, MORE! Thus, what was once an easy basic became a fraught style statement with its own internal fashion trends.

The style that originally reeled in the masses was the bootcut hipster. The hipster jean was clever because it differentiated jeans from the high-waisted yokel versions of old, thereby justifying their three-figure price tag. The bootcut was a little trickier. The theory behind this style is that by widening out the ankle, the thigh will look proportionally slimmer. There is some merit in this, but, really, you have to wonder about the intelligence of any onlooker who thinks, "Wow, look how that lady's ankles seem to be about the same width as her thighs—golly, her thighs must be as thin as reeds! Hubba, hubba!" The fact is, your thighs are still visible, so it is an optical illusion with a brief life span. If you really want to disguise your thighs, then you're going to have to wear wide-legged jeans and deal with the fact that you now resemble an extra in *On the Town*. Moreover, by beginning to widen out the cut midway down your calf, you are merely truncating the apparent length of your legs, which surely goes against the ultimate selling point of most jeans and their much-vaunted leg-lengthening properties. Bootcut is still the most flattering denim style for most people. But make no mistake, you are wearing denim flares, a style some of us thought we'd never see again outside of documentary Woodstock footage.

Yet it was overexposure that began to turn the fashion tide against the once seemingly almighty bootcut style. Because of its convenience and promises of instant slimness, it became as associated with yummy mummies as Bugaboos and daytime yoga classes. And so, as always happens with a fashion trend, an alternative was needed—though it was an alternative few thought would succeed: *et voilà,* the era of the skinny jean.

The skinny jean is manna from the fashion gods (or H&M, anyway), if you like to wear your boots over your jeans and check your cellulite without removing any clothes. What it's not so great for is anyone over a size 6. Just as "bootcut" is just a fancy-pants word for "flared," so "skinny jeans" is just a euphemism for "denim leggings," a style that didn't even make it in the '80s.

But thanks to Kate Moss looking good in them (see **Moss, Kate, and how she ruined your wardrobe**) and to bootcut exhaustion, skinny jeans were as ubiquitous as James Blunt for some time. But just because something has the word "skinny" in the name does not mean it will actually make you skinny. If anything, you could see it as operating like an NC-17 rating on a film, in that it describes the only people who are advised to partake.

Men seem to understand this, so you see them wearing skinny jeans only if they're musicians, who subsist on a diet of opium and groupies, or half-starved fashion students. Women, however, are a more optimistic, or maybe just more self-confident breed and happily squeeze themselves into the tightest denim leggings they can buy.

Some find this blatant show of female curvature aesthetically upsetting. Yeah, well, some people apparently still take Tom Cruise seriously—what can you do about it? The real problem with skinny jeans is that they quietly ushered in their inevitable descendant, leggings, the non-denim kind. Because women had gotten used to wearing something super-tight on their legs with a normal top, they felt comfortable pairing leggings with a hip- or waist-length top. Now, as lovely as a woman's anatomy is, there is no need to confront the general public with her gusset. It was certainly an interesting spin on the '80s look of leggings with a long top, but there are times when you have to ask yourself if there is a reason this style didn't work in the decade in which it originated.

Like bootcut, the hipster element was also ripe for a fall from grace because of its similar ubiquity, and so in 2005 and 2006 various brands dabbled with high-waisted styles, pish-tushing aside any complaints that this would remind people of how unflattering jeans once were. The thing about high-waisted is that although it will make you look thinner from the back because it pinches in your waist and holds in muffin topage—a common problem with hipster jeans—it's generally not the same story from the front and sides. All the flesh that's being pinched in will be forced downwards to give you a denim pregnant bump. This can be quite a useful shelf on which to rest things like mugs of tea, but some people might feel this doesn't compensate for its various disadvantages.

All of these issues illustrate why one should never pay attention to trends when it comes to trousers. Trends exist to allow customers to skip gaily through the fields of novelty, dabbling with different looks, like small children let loose in the dress-up cupboard. I'm afraid trousers are just too serious a matter to be treated so frivolously. Because they hug and emphasize very particular parts of one's anatomy, it is easy to look terrible in them or, arguably more important, just to feel uncomfortable in them. Find the style that suits you best and, come hell or high water, cling to it firmly. No one particular style suits everyone; anyone who tells you different is trying to sell you something.

Jeans' colors have gone through a similar new-and-improved to ironic-and-retro trajectory. At first, it was the most flattering shade, dark blue, but this quickly became dull and, with the emergence of the phenomenally successful 7 For All Mankind jeans, this then moved to lighter blue to faded gray to black to, most improbably of all, white. Well, at least Elizabeth Hurley is happy, but then, she does have to live on watercress soup to fit into them, which might temper one's feelings of envy.

Feathering and bleaching became popular and annoying design tweaks. Why anyone thought creased white lines in the crotch area would add appeal to anything is beyond me. Feathering basically makes you look like your geriatric merkin has slipped out of place or that you have drawn some helpful arrows pointing the, um, way. As for fading, jeans fade because the denim wears down from being stretched over your body. It's odd that someone would want to buy jeans that look like they have been so worn down from trying to rein in her heft. Moreover, the fading is always over the front of the legs and the bum, precisely the areas that work better with darker colors, not giant bleach spots magnifying them like spotlights.

The most flattering jeans I ever owned were a pair of simple, dark blue, straight-legged Earl jeans that sat just below the hip but high enough so I could sit without looking like I was ready for my colonic, bought back in the days when the word "iPod" looked more like the name of a Teletubby than a daily necessity. Now they hark back to a simpler, nobler time and, not to come over all *Wonder Years* on you, things really were much better then. No question, jeans needed some improving. But when manufacturers started making solemn statements about light blue being this year's faded gray and knocking out limited-edition, crystal-studded $600 jeans, the denim industry jumped the shark. Jeans became so popular only because retailers learned how to make them look good. So to then start knocking out high-waisted versions in white does suggest that sight of their original appeal has been well and truly lost. But it's not just retailers who are to blame; once something becomes too popular, we, the consumers, get bored and move on to a previously untapped style. Yet the reason that style—white jeans, say—has not been seized yet by the masses is because it's not all that hot. Thus, in a scenario that recalls the film *Sophie's Choice*, you have to choose sometimes between looking fashionable and looking good. Your decision, but just ask yourself what you'd rather spend money on—impressing the overgrown kids in a bar in Brooklyn or looking so fabulous you briefly consider having sex with your reflection in the bathroom mirror. No wonder so many people began to opt out and run to the simpler embrace of shorts with tights and, sigh, leggings.

So there we go—we learned how to make the perfect jeans and then we went and put a wrench in the whole process. Ah well, you can't have everything. After all, as British comedian Steve Wright once so wisely pointed out, where would you put it?

Jewelry, and when fashion just gets obnoxious

A Venn diagram showing where the fur customer and the jewelry customer overlap is merely one giant circle. As with fur, you can just about see the appeal of super-expensive jewelry: it's shiny and twinkly and occasionally sort of pretty. So are fairy lights, but that doesn't mean I'm going to spend $100,000 on them. Ultimately, it's just a quick way to flash some serious cash that, unlike fur, doesn't have the faint justification of keeping you warm. There is absolutely no point to real jewelry except to show off how rich you are and divert thieves from the rest of us poor folk. Perhaps if you were living in some soon-to-be-toppled economy and had to convert your remaining life savings into something that wouldn't be worthless by tomorrow, jewelry would make more sense. Seeing as few readers are currently living in early-twentieth-century Russia, that argument holds little sway around here. You know the facts: it's offensively expensive; the gems are often unearthed by distastefully unethical methods involving small children and underground caves;

and if you don't feel disgusted at wearing something that costs more than what most people spend on a down payment for a house, then it might be time to do a little bit of soul-searching. Wedding rings—fine; earrings to celebrate something like a tenth anniversary—fine; flashy jewelry for the sake of looking good at the latest charity dinner for whatever this month's trendy benefit is—not cool. Just give the charity the money you spent on that stupid brooch that makes you look like you dribbled on your lapel, you daft woman, you.

Of course, not all jewelry makes one come over like a rampaging communist. Just don't go too far with it simply to show off. A sure way of knowing when you've done this is when you get out the "Statement Piece." Think oversized clanging earrings, think hideous brooches, think whacking great necklaces dangling down a woman's cleavage, and you've pretty much got the idea.

There are several problems with statement jewelry. First, it does precisely what it says on the can—it makes a statement—and that statement tends to be that this oversized brooch in the shape of a bunch of gladioli is all you have to offer to the fashion conversation today. Moreover, it suggests that you are very proud of this piece, and you might want to think twice before saying that about a gladioli brooch. And finally, because you're metaphorically and possibly literally shoving it in people's faces, everyone will, if only out of politeness, comment on it throughout the day, and you will have to trot out the story about how your grandmother left it to you in her will or whatever at least fifteen times, depending on how popular you are and how polite your friends are, until the sound of your own voice will make you want to rip that pin out of your lapel and stab it in your vocal cords. And speaking of politeness, here's a handy hint: if you hear the sentence, usually uttered in a tone best described as "tremulous," "Oooh, what an extraordinary pin, wherever did you get it?" this should be taken as a decorous euphemism rather than a compliment. And if you hear it more than three times in twenty-four hours, ditch the pin.

But, to quote the name of an old '80s book from this author's childhood, *Jewelry Can Be Fun!* And, in fact, that's when it's at its best—being fun and not all po-faced and ostentatious. Moreover, if it's a half-decent party, you are guaranteed to lose at least one piece of jewelry so it just makes better sense to get, say, a $30 necklace in the shape of a chunky heart than a $300,000 pink diamond ring. *Sex and the City* was quite the master at this, showing how a woman can take pleasure in jewelry without it

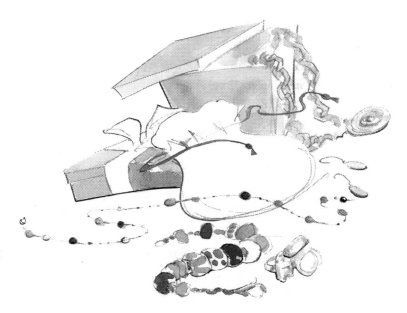

descending into kitsch or clownish territory, such as Carrie's multistranded necklace of fake pearls and pretty dangling earrings. (The nameplate necklace went too far. Who goes around flaunting their name in a big city, anyway?) Long earrings are certainly a lot more fun than boring preppy studs; oversized fake cocktail rings work with both jeans and T-shirts or party outfits and cost at most $20; long swinging strands of necklaces can look good, but you have to be flat-chested, as otherwise they look like a topographical chart of a local hilly area. Brooches are completely pointless: in what way does sticking some gimmicky little image in your lapel add to an outfit? Oversized hoop earrings had their moment until everyone realized that having one's lobes dragged down by the weight of these hoops or, worse, ripped downward when their fingers got caught in them while doing a flirtatious hair-flick really did not help a lady's mood on a night out. If you want a simple analogy, think of it like this: accessories are the sprinkles on a cake, there to improve, not form the whole meal. They are not essential and, when done badly, are cloying. But when employed with a sage and delicate hand, they make the difference between generic blandness and decorative indulgence.

Lagerfeld, Karl, and why he's so brilliant

There are many reasons to love Karl Lagerfeld, but number one has got to be because—and this is meant in truly the best, most respectful of ways—he is such a fantastic bitch. His *mots*, some *bons* but more usually downright *mauvais,* are infamous, not just because of their perceptive accuracy but because of the way he says them with a guileless, even supportive, expression, when in fact he may as well be carving out your heart with a spoon.

When Chanel dropped Kate Moss after the cocaine "shock" scandal, only to realize that, actually, the public wasn't quite as hypocritical as the media, Lagerfeld praised her for having "a lot of courage in the way she throws her life away in a very dangerous way, but that makes her so touching." This is he being nice, by the way. Most famously, when Chloé hired Stella McCartney to take over as the brand's creative director, Lagerfeld said, calm as you like, "I guess they wanted a name. Unfortunately, they chose one in music, not fashion." Yet, incredibly, despite the bitchiness, Lagerfeld has managed to construct the most extraordinary self-image of being some ascetic intellectual, someone who scorns fashion fripperies to go home and read Proust in Aramaic before whipping off another thirty drawings for his next collection, rereading the whole of Emily Dickinson, and then putting his priceless art collection in chronological order. And how do we know he does this? Because he constantly tells us. As self-branding methods go, it's not the most subtle. He talks loudly of how he hates most people (fair enough), has never taken drugs (probably true), and has no interest in sex (who knows? who wants to?). Even though almost all autobiographical details he has ever uttered have proven to be total baloney, from his aristocratic German childhood, oddly untouched by the Nazis, to whether or not he's ever been in love, the view of Lagerfeld as some sexless, inhuman genius still seems to be the generally accepted one. Recently, a German tabloid managed to confront him with incontrovertible proof of his wariness of a concept called the truth by unearthing his birth certificate, showing that Lagerfeld is actually a few years older than he had always claimed. Lagerfeld, proving that he does have previously denied cojones, responded by saying he would never reply to such "trash." This coming from a man who once dubbed Lindsay Lohan "an icon" really is something.

His physical appearance also merits commendation. Once he was a ponytailed butterball who hid behind a fan to "block out other people's bad breath." But then one morning he decided he didn't like that look so much anymore. Instead, he wanted to wear trousers made by his tango-dancing partner (and that is not, all parties insist, a euphemism), Hedi Slimane, formerly at Dior Homme. And so, on a diet he claims consisted primarily of cactus juice, this sixty/seventy-something managed to lose over 80 pounds. Now he looks like a psychotic sixteenth-century German courtier, just as he'd intended.

Another reason to love him is that, rather sweetly, the only time he makes good clothes is when he makes them in someone else's name. Lagerfeld's clothes for Chloé? Adorable, beautiful, splendid. His clothes for Chanel? Iconic, unbeatable, up there with the best in the world. His clothes for Fendi? Well, they're great, if you like that skinned-chinchilla-coat look, which apparently a lot of people do. His clothes for his own label, Karl Lagerfeld? Not such winners. You didn't even know they existed, did you? And what must really grate is that Lagerfeld subscribes to the Donatella Versace approach to fashion in making the collection in his own image. Thus, should you accidentally find yourself at a Lagerfeld fashion show, you will more likely than not be confronted with a parade of thirty models all looking exactly like Lagerfeld, with slicked-back hair and scary *Matrix-*

like suits. When a sixty- (or seventy-) something-year-old German designer is able to make an eighteen-year-old girl from San Francisco look like him, you know you are dealing with a serious talent. Sadly, few people actually want to look like a pensionable German designer. But Lagerfeld, of course, claims not to give a damn.

His clothes for Chanel, in particular, really are fantastic. They manage to stay on just the right side of pastiche so that they are recognizably Chanel without looking as if you're en route to a costume party. They keep the original Chanel appeal—ladylike but girlish, a little bit cool but very proper—and make it modern: delicate dresses mixed with biker boots or piles of charm necklaces over a tweed jacket. It is hard to think of many other designers who can appeal to Sofia Coppola, Paris Hilton, and Lauren Bacall in a single collection. Perhaps the only other one who can do this is Marc Jacobs (see **Jacobs, Marc: genius or what?**), who has publicly stated that his dream gig would be to take over at Chanel, only for Lagerfeld to turn around and publicly state, more or less, that Jacobs could go boil his head.

Lagerfeld treats everything as a costume. He has adopted some weird personae, maybe just because he wanted to, but almost certainly because he knew that such extremism would bring him fame, and that is often the best advertisement for the brand. If he were really so private, we wouldn't know about it; if he were really such an effete intellectual snob, he wouldn't bring Lindsay Lohan as his date to a fashion dinner. Everything is about creating a perfectly constructed image, whether it be speaking total nonsense about his childhood or living on cactus juice; no wonder he flounders when it comes to designing his own collection. For this reason, he is the perfect designer for these image-obsessed days. Though if he ever heard this kind of psychoanalysis, he would probably tell me to choke on it. And Karl, I'd love you even more for that.

Late, fashionably, and just rude

It is unfortunate that the word "late" has somehow adopted adverb "fashionably," thereby fixing and perpetuating the idea in the collective mind that it is elegant to keep people waiting. It is not. It is annoying and is yet another example of the irritating teenage mentality that pervades many areas of the fashion industry. Legends of lateness abound in the industry, the most famous probably being that of Naomi Campbell, who once allegedly turned up right on the hour the fashion shoot was scheduled to start, albeit three days after the agreed date.

When you are late, you are basically saying that your time is more important than that of the person you're meant to meet, which you may well believe, but it does seem a bit harsh to rub their noses in it for the thirty minutes they sit waiting for you. When fashion people are late, they are insinuating that they lead such glamorous, busy lives, jetting from Diddy in Malibu to Tom Ford in London, that people are lucky to get them at all. Thus, it is a very handy kind of self-advertisement, though one that will make most people hate you.

And the truth is, most fashion people do know this. They do know that turning up to meetings late is perhaps not the most professional way to behave and, in fact, no way to run a business. Thus, the dirty truth is that—shhhh!—most fashion people aren't late at all. Yes, it's true: designers don't tend to turn up half an hour late to interviews with journalists, and publicists are generally bang on time for those crucial expense lunches with editors. But this is something people like to keep quiet about as it's just not very cool. The only time they all are late is when everyone's on display for one another, i.e., at fashion shows and parties. Tellingly, the one person who is never late to either of these crucial events is Anna Wintour, who is always to be found perched in the front row, dead on time at the shows, even though she knows she will have to spend at least the next hour staring blankly ahead from behind her sunglasses without even a newspaper to help her while away the time (props to alleviate boredom are, it seems, somehow even less cool than being on time). As I said, this is telling because it proves that this lateness malarkey really is just about convincing everyone of your importance, and if there is one person in this industry who does not need to bother to do this, it is Wintour, seeing as she is the big kahuna of the whole shebang. It is somehow even more telling that being on time is possibly the one trend that Wintour has not been able to convince her followers to adopt. Yeah, well, we are talking about looking cool here, and even Anna's powers can extend only so far.

Layering, the whats and the hows of

The line between looking stylishly layered and appearing residentially challenged is a slender one. But then, the line between the patron saint of layering, Kurt Cobain, and a homeless man wasn't exactly fat either.

Matters aren't helped by fashion shoots involving models

dashing around country piles wearing all manner of silk slip dresses and heavy tweed coats and anoraks that purport to show how glamorous layering can be but, in fact, to the untrained eye, look more like documentary footage from a 1930s lunatic asylum.

Fashion magazines love the layering look because it appears so devil-may-care in that uniquely aristo way, and they can get something from every single advertiser into one shoot. Designers love it because it makes people think that instead of buying just one sweater they should buy three, an oversized blouse, a skirt, and maybe those extra-thick socks, too. Whether either of these factors was what Kurt intended is unknown, but it is not for us to fathom the mind of a genius.

All you need to know about layering is that it is a handy way to stay warm. Thus, long-sleeved shirts can go under summer dresses, and woolly tights have been shown to work surprisingly well under delicate party dresses. A pretty camisole over a long-sleeved shirt is just about acceptable, but prepare yourself to be asked by your father whether you're off to battle in your new suit of armor—hilarious! So keep it simple and no more than two or, at a push, three items at a time. This is what a trend should do: reveal ways to wear clothes you never considered and in ways you can continue to wear them for more than the present six months, such as summer dresses over thin-knit sweaters. It should not be about brainwashing people into wearing something so laughably stupid that they spend the rest of their lives tracking down photos of themselves from that era in order to destroy them.

For boys, the situation is subtly different, simply because they have a longer and not entirely noble layering tradition that has, therefore, picked up all manner of associations. Of course, the faux stoner look grates as the wearer, trying to go for a laid-back California dude effect, is clearly as image-conscious as your average socialite. Piling a T-shirt on top of a long-sleeved top is not a dressing ritual that comes naturally. Unless, of course, he *is* stoned, which at least explains why he doesn't seem to have washed either of the tops since 1998.

Even more wearying is a single, articulated garment made to give a double layered effect. Like pre-ripped jeans, pre-washed trousers, or pre-bleached T-shirts, this is the worst kind of lazy artificiality, up there with pre-chipped "antique" wooden furniture from a department store or a "homemade" Entenmann's chocolate cake. This is not to say that we should all return to making our own bread or whatever, because we all know that ready-made is generally a lot better—well, a lot easier, anyway, which down my way amounts to the same thing. But if you are going to embrace the artificial, at least acknowledge that, rather than pretending you're really communing with nature with your genuine replica Apothecary Table from Pottery Barn. And if you really are too lazy to layer two shirts on top of one another yourself, well then, maybe that is God's way of telling you that you shouldn't bother.

Leather jackets, and the delusion of the middle-aged man

Ah, Bruce Springsteen, Paul Weller, and Joe Strummer. The havoc that you have wreaked! You thought you were expressing the primal male psyche; in fact, you provided the fashion template for men to express that beneath a Brooks Brothers button-down shirt beats the heart of a young tiger, whose legs are metaphorically slung over a motorcycle on Route 66 even if, in reality, they are squeezed inside a Honda Civic on car pool duty.

Just as skinny jeans often emphasize the distance between fantasy and reality, so does dressing in clothes from one's youth. In fact, the yawning gap between seventeen and fifty-five yawns wider in the contrast between the leather collar and the gravity-embracing jowls. We should all salute the power of fashion and all that, but a leather jacket is not Marty McFly's DeLorean. Just get yourself a decent woolen jacket or even a smart wool or tweed coat and be done with it. It's a little like when celebrities claim, despite all visible evidence, that they are twenty-six. Yet the general public are not quite so stupid, and aren't going to nod their heads and bovinely repeat as one, "Twenty-six, yes, mistress, you are twenty-six . . ." Instead, those who aren't raising their eyebrows in awe at the audacity of the celebrity's ploy will merely muse on how old the celebrity looks for her age and how badly she seems to be aging, poor thing. Claiming to be twenty-six won't make you look twenty-six, any more than forcing yourself into a pair of size 4 trousers will make you look like a size 4; and dressing like Bruce won't fool people into thinking you were, indeed, born to run, in your Honda Civic, if need be.

Limits, age, and what's (allegedly) acceptable when

Alongside "the new elegance" and "what's hot now," the most popular fashion magazine coverline is "how to look fabulous at every age" or variations thereof. It is notable how this idea is invariably touted as a revelation: my God, can you actually imagine a woman looking good past the age of thirty-five? The answer, more common than not, is no, not if you pay any attention to the advice inside the magazine.

And no surprise, really. Designers are frequently accused of taking a harder line against age than the folk in *Logan's Run*. In truth, though, designers have some respect for a more mature vintage, if only because it tends to comprise a large proportion of their customer base. There are only so many Paris Hiltons to go around, you know, and even in that case I'd wager Paris's mother has access to a bigger Visa account.

The confusion comes from the fact that these grannyish tweed jackets and professional businesswoman suits are invariably modeled by sunken-cheeked barely pubescents. And who decides that this is how the system must work? The magazines. Sure, the designers might use these underweight children in their shows, but a show lasts only five minutes twice a year, and maybe that doesn't give designers long enough to realize how ridiculous it looks to have a catwalk full of little girls who appear to have just emerged from their grandmother's closet. Magazines, however, do this every day, all year long, and the lesson has yet to sink in. So why should anyone expect them to know what looks good on a sixty-five-year-old, seeing as they insist on dressing eighteen-year-olds in clothes for someone who's fifty years old?

Anyway, the usual rubric of fashion magazine features is to have one photo of a (very young) model for each decade, in which the passage of time is generally marked by a growing penchant for blazers and increasingly ornate accessories to "give you a bit of sparkle"—something which apparently diminishes with age.

Many rules get bandied about concerning what's acceptable in which decade—wide-legged trousers, good; sleeveless tops, bad—all of which can be summed up in one sentence: the older you are, the less of you we want to see. Some people in the West might reel back in horror at the Muslim tradition of making women wear burkas to hide their unacceptable femininity, but moral superiority seems misplaced when we do the same thing, albeit slightly later and using more expensive labels.

The biggest concern of these features is to teach women what is "appropriate" for their age, and, over the age of forty, showing skin at all is "inappropriate" because someone, somewhere, might see skin that isn't entirely smooth. The horror, the horror!

Of course, as one gets older, one's body changes, and what once looked cute might start to merit a different adjective. But the reason women dress too young for their age is that they understandably fear being dismissed by the anti-over-thirty-five culture. It seems unlikely that counseling them to wear blazers with brass buttons and carrying "sparkly" handbags will make them feel better about the future. The circles are vicious.

In truth, the real fault in dressing too young for your age is not the aesthetic distress it might cause onlookers. Rather, it suggests that you have failed to learn certain lessons over the years. Only the very young, for example, are (just about) tolerated for wearing T-shirts with silly slogans, simply because their brains are still soft and have yet to soak in the lesson that this is not the last word in chic. The twenties and early thirties are a hard time of life, when one begins to realize that Saturday night is no longer synonymous with getting smashed out of your brain but rather is the reality of dithering over a Nigella Lawson cookbook, while your friends sit in the living room talking about things like mortgages and child care. No wonder these traumatized souls so frequently try to block out the roar of encroaching maturity by buying overpriced accessories. By the time a lady is in her forties, she probably is beginning to emerge from this cocoon of trend dabbling and showing herself to be the butterfly she always was, now aware of what suits her and what doesn't. Once she reaches her fifties, she knows that wearing high heels all day long is absurd, and that wide-legged trousers and flats are actually far better propositions than those magazines let on (particularly when paired with a cool, short-sleeved blouse). And by the time she gets into her sixties—well, it would be downright insulting for me to make any suggestions, as now she is far too wise to need any guidance in this department, having long since found the style that suits her.

This issue of personal style is utterly jettisoned by features about age. Just as horoscopes seem to believe that a twelfth of the population will be making a journey on a given day, simply because they were all born in early May, so these articles operate on the idea that whole age groups have exactly the same personal tastes, figures, and forms of self-expression. Maybe some Taureans are going on a journey that day, and maybe some sixty-somethings genuinely do long for an Armani trouser suit. But I'd wager many aren't and don't.

The fashion magazines protest that they're giving women confidence because they show how one can look good as one gets older, despite the fact that, um, they've been saying the opposite for the rest of the year. And this would be a reasonable argument if it didn't have a touch of the brainwashing cult leader to it: "Come, follow our way, never mind your own personal inclinations." As I said, some women do dress too young for their age, to no one's benefit, but there is a world of alternatives between a pink ruffled party dress and a boring blue trouser suit.

And if a woman manages to get to the unimaginably ancient age of, say, fifty-two without having been bludgeoned into hermit-hood or turned into a raving fanatic by the bias toward youth, well, I'd say she has more than earned the right to wear a sleeveless top if she darn well wishes.

Lingerie, and the importance or otherwise of an audience

When Andrea Dworkin was out there fighting for women to take control of their bodies and their sexuality, she probably didn't consider how brilliantly her principles would relate to the lingerie business. Nor is it likely that her secret life's ambition was to see her name in a fashion book, in a section about lingerie. But, as Dworkin has no doubt mused somewhere, we live in an era when a woman's destiny is still not wholly in her power.

Once sexy lingerie was all about the audience; the wearer was forced to truss herself up in nasty, itchy stuff that probably had a detachable bunny tail. But then a nice couple called Joe Corre and Serena Rees came up with the idea that looking sexy and feeling uncomfortable need not be quite so closely aligned. Lo, Agent Provocateur was born, teaching the world that "sexy lingerie" wasn't French for "red and scratchy."

The thing is, while it is always nice to be appreciated, lingerie should be about making the wearer feel good herself. Forget about G-strings, which are horrible and make no woman feel sexy, unless "sexy" has somehow become a synonym for "two molars, mid-floss" (see **G-strings, and the female lie**). But it is very cheering during another dull day in the office to know that you have pretty little satin things with bits of frills here and there beneath your crumpled suit.

Some women say they find it depressing to wear nice lingerie without the prospect of an audience. Yeah, well, some women actually watched *Ally McBeal* instead of dismissing it for the misogynistic twaddle it was. To see lingerie as a spectator sport is to miss the point of fashion—to make yourself feel good—and to play right into the hands of all those who scold women, saying fashion is shallow and vain (and all of you silly girls should get back into your frumpy old sack dresses and into the kitchen where you belong). And so, as Andrea would no doubt say if she were still here, "Go on, ladies, fight against misogynists: go out there and buy some silk knickers!" Yeah! Right on!

Logos: the bleating of the insecure

One might have thought that it would be difficult to put a price on the inner glow of validation. Oh naïveté! It's an easy 150 percent markup, madam, and have a nice day. Designer logos are a reassuring pat on the head to those who are so devoid of any confidence in their own taste that they rely on the name of someone they've never met, and probably wouldn't even like, to be slapped on their clothes and accessories to reassure them they've made a good purchase. This also means that the man or woman sporting the logo has such low expectations of their fellow human creatures that they expect them, too, to be impressed by this billboard look, which, when you think about it, is kind of insulting. Really, it's surprising that fashion companies spend billions of dollars every year on magazine advertising when so many customers out there are happy to pay them to do it for them.

Louis Vuitton must be the prime culprit on this score, not because the line necessarily slaps its name about more than anyone else (Chanel, Dior, and Armani could easily give it a run for its money, and that's not even mentioning Burberry's plaid, Missoni's stripes, or Pucci's swirls, which serve pretty much the same purpose as a logo) but because it has milked so much more out of this wheeze. Louis Vuitton luggage and handbags are little more than well made but irrefutably dull brown suitcases. Yet because of that tan LV motif adorning the hardware, they not only cost more than most pieces of furniture but also have somehow become an indisputable symbol of French chic. Vuitton's creative director, Marc Jacobs, has enjoyed huge success by having a bit of fun with this logo veneration thing, and by "fun" I mean making them multicolored, decorating them with Japanese cartoon flowers, and turning them into graffiti tags. Some might describe this as ironic; others might see it as proof that all the guff about Louis Vuitton has less to do with the logo's oft-cited "timeless appeal" and rather more to do with the timeless desire to flaunt designer names.

I'm all for people getting credit where credit's due, and one could say that a designer logo works in the same way as do credits at the end of a film. Yet film credits tend to come quietly at the end of the movie; they aren't splattered across the film itself.

Once you have a name that is deemed worthy of becoming a logo, you pretty much have a license to print money. Stick it on a plastic compact that probably cost about seven cents to manufacture and flog the silly thing for forty bucks; slosh it across the backs of jeans, bikinis, and even ski equipment if you like, and multiply the retail price tags by at least three. Ah, there's nothing like being in the fresh alpine air, looking down at one's feet, and seeing the reassuring double C of the Chanel logo on your skis to really make you feel you're connecting with nature.

Aside from the garishness of logos and the fact that they add several zeros to price tags and then scream this fact to onlookers, they reek of the worst kind of fashion victimhood. They suggest such an obsequious mentality: "This dress is hideous. Oh wait a minute, it says 'Lacroix' across the front, so it must be okay." They reduce fashion itself to its most cynical cliché—that it is merely conspicuous consumption—rather than a venue of self-expression. If you can only justify the purchase by the fact that someone else's name is written across it as opposed to, say, its simple beauty, then it's probably not a purchase worth making. Heck, you may as well just buy a ten-cent name tag from Office

Depot, write a designer's name on that, and pin it to yourself. And if your sense of self is dependent on walking around wearing someone else's name, well, some soul searching might be the order of the day.

Logos more than any other style statement are glaringly dependent on context, which is why designers get all in a fluster when the "wrong sort" sport them. When an acceptably aspirational A-lister flaunts them, she—the general mentality goes—looks rich and glamorous. But when someone a little lower down on the celebrity alphabet wears the same, logos are shown up for what they are: the bleating of the insecure, desperate for acceptance by the chronically shallow. In this sense, they are a useful reminder of how thumpingly useless it is to look to fashion icons for style guidance (see **Celebrities, and when bad ones happen to good fashion**). In all other respects, they are the detritus of a look that should have faded out with the heydey of Ivana Trump.

Low-slung belts, and the point thereof

Not a lot, one would have thought. And one would be right. Some people, bless their souls, think that a belt is meant to hold up your pants. They are still mentally operating in the pre-Sienna era, that time before a blond West Londoner showed how putting on an oversized belt made one look thinner (Look, I'm so thin even my belt can't fit around my childlike hips!), cooler (I am so busy, dashing between my A-list boyfriend and my private plane to Marrakech, that I don't even have time to put my belt on properly!), and pleasingly eco-aware, thanks to its vaguely hippie connotations.

To be fair, a low-slung belt can help to control the potential maternity-sack look of that new tunic dress you bought from Gap by gently reining in its volume, whereas a normal belt would cinch your waist and stomach, thereby divesting the tunic of its main appeal—that you can eat as much as you like in it without looking like a snake digesting a rabbit. Plus, it does give an interesting insight into what it must feel like to be a teenage boy who insists on wearing his jeans halfway down around his upper thighs (answer: quite stupid and a little incapacitated), and it's always nice to show a little empathy with the lower forms of life. But in all other instances, it is gratingly superfluous.

Magazines, fashion, and women's masochistic love thereof

The argument that fashion makes women feel bad about themselves can be disproved by one little number: 1.3 million. That's how many copies of *Vogue* are read in the U.S. every month. And while a certain portion of those readers may well be whip wielders and bondage queens, I'd be surprised if they accounted for the total. The idea that women are meekly buying *InStyle* every month in order to punish themselves has the suspicious stench of a ready-made theory reheated by lazy newspaper columnists with a word count to fill and a deadline to meet.

We now live in an era when most of us dose ourselves up with more drugs at the first hint of a cold than Syd Barrett got through in a week, buy pre-chopped vegetables to save a whole two minutes' cooking time, and do a large part of our shopping over the Internet, thereby brilliantly avoiding inconveniences such as standing up and walking. So the idea that women would go out of their way to find something to make life hard for themselves doesn't have the smack of likelihood. The truth is, women buy fashion magazines because they like them. Fashion magazines full of pretty girls wearing expensive clothes and living ever so glamorous lives should make you feel no worse about yourself than, say, some high-octane blockbuster film full of, ahem, pretty girls wearing expensive clothes and living their own glamorous (multiorgasmic) lives, but I have yet to hear anyone take Harvey Weinstein to task for women's mental health the way they have Anna Wintour. Magazines, like movies, are there to provide you with a few hours of fantasy fun; that's why women buy them. If they were templates for reality, they'd be called life magazines, not fashion magazines, and, as we can all see reality every day for free, they'd probably have a much lower circulation.

If a woman is already prone to self-hatred, then, yes, she will find a fair amount of fodder to nurture those tendencies in a fashion magazine, just as she would at her local multiplex. For the majority, sure, maybe there is some initial self-dissatisfaction when looking at pages of hipless women, overpriced dresses, and holidays that are about as close to most people's reality as a day in the life of James Bond. But this ill-feeling is swiftly dissipated by the sheer fun of looking at the clothes, picking out the ones you'd buy in a parallel universe—and finding similar versions in H&M—and reading another article about high hems written with the kind of solemnity reserved for think tank reports. Women, by and large, are not small children incapable of distinguishing between fantasy and reality; even if a woman were to spend five solid years reading a fashion magazine, there is no guarantee that she would come away thinking that jutting bones and piano-key ribs are the norm. She might have a slightly skewed perception of good value when it comes to clothes, but that's a different issue.

You want to know another reason women buy fashion magazines? Because sometimes it's nice to read something that is just for us. Not about our kids, not about our boyfriends—and how to "please" them—not about our jobs, or our parents, or about any worthwhile cultural or political issue we know we should understand better, but 100 percent about us. Not us in reality, of course, but us in a fantasy world, where we get fresh sea salt scrubs in Bali every "spring break," whatever that is, and actually do revamp our entire wardrobes every six months. It's a land where your ShopRite bag never splits in the middle of the street, where boyfriends never dump you, and where you never spend another night watching another day in the life of *Grey's Anatomy*. We just want lots of lovely pictures of things we could wear and interviews with people who "divide their time" between multiple continents.

Moreover, because they can't criticize anything (see **Advertising: how it spins the fashion axis**), fashion magazines are decidedly upbeat affairs. They are certainly far more cheerful than the weekly gossip magazines that have sprouted like fungi in the past five years. These are almost entirely comprised of allegedly bad photos of female celebrities who have dared to be mid-blink when the shutter clicked or left the house in something other than Dior couture, the shameless slatterns. These magazines like to claim that bringing celebrities down a peg makes women feel better, when, really, their message is that a woman must never blink when a camera's in the room, as even Uma Thurman gets scolded about this.

In the land of the fashion magazine, however, everyone is fabulous and no one ever does anything wrong. Admittedly, the increasingly prevalent interviews with eighteen-year-old models can be a bit of a downer, purely due to their uniformity: favorite food—sushi; favorite pastime—surfing, sure as eggs, every time. Still, it's nice to have something you can rely on in this cold world of ours.

And even if the magazine isn't up to its usual snuff one month and doesn't provide you with the usual satisfaction, the knowledge that there are 1.3 million other *Grey's Anatomy* escapists out there probably will.

Makeup: the tears of a clown

Like high heels, makeup is one of those things that cause you to simultaneously pity and envy the male of the species. Pity because one has to be occasionally grateful for armory at a lady's service, but envy, too, because it is a bit of a pain to be expected to put this extensive armory to use instead of just slinging oneself in the shower, spritzing on a bit of CK aftershave, and heading out on the town, confident that one has done about as much as one is reasonably expected to do.

There is something slightly odd in the idea of makeup, anyway. With its emphasis on colored eyelids, unnaturally heavy lashes, pink cheeks, and big red lips, one cannot but trace a very obvious lineage between a gal's nighttime look and that of a clown. Sure, slightly flushed cheeks and pinked lips might make one look a little nicer on washed-out days, even if, inevitably, some wiseass somewhere has propounded the theory that the appeal of this is that it makes a woman look, yes, mid-orgasm (see also **Heels: the highs, the lows, and when fat is better than thin** for a similar theory that suggests that sociocultural theorists spend too many sweaty-palmed hours in the library). And we've all had cause to thank the little guy who invented concealer.

Yes, makeup does make us look better, or what our view of "better" is. Most of the time this means simply "younger" (see **Antiaging**) or "a little less tired." But without wishing to come across as too ragingly militant here, perhaps we need to reconsider some of our concepts of beauty, because there are some cosmetics that make neither hide nor hair of sense. Colored eyelids, anyone? Just who decided that neon-colored eyelids were the surest way to a man's heart, or simply a fast track to a party look in general? Curling eyelashes are, to be honest, just weird, and eye pencil as a whole is an odd concept, at least to anyone who has a natural aversion to sticking a pencil into their eyeball or giving themselves catlike eyes with a marker pen. Lip liner is a no-win idea, because either your lips have a naturally defined line already or, if it is slightly faded because of "feathering," also known as wrinkles, the liner will often emphasize this by falling into the, um, feathers, or whatever the accepted euphemistic term is. Lip gloss is great if you actively pursue the "mouth slobberer" look and find trying to talk with strands of hair attached to your lips a welcome challenge. And don't even get me started on red fingernails. All right, fine, do: excellent if you want to look like some Agatha Christie murderer, blood dripping from your fingers. Once you ask yourself why some things are prized above others, veritable floodgates open that may, admittedly, say more about your own psyche than that of society's.

Anything that will give you what the beauty industry calls, with its endearing obliviousness to the concept of the oxymoron, a "natural sparkle" is permissible only if you are still not legally allowed to buy alcohol or if you have somehow jumped back in time and turned up in Studio 54, circa 1978.

Unless you are a burlesque dancer, makeup is generally there to make you look better, not make you look like you're wearing makeup. Hence, "the 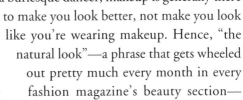 natural look"—a phrase that gets wheeled out pretty much every month in every fashion magazine's beauty section— basically means a full face of makeup but the lips perhaps a little more pink than full-on red and the eyelashes slightly longer and darker. "The vamp look," on the other hand, is pleasingly honest in its description because, with its inevitably powdered face, pruned-back eyebrows, and crimson lips, it does encapsulate how most people imagine a vampire to look. No one is really sure what on earth the "preppy" and "English rose" looks really mean, other than, in both cases, an appreciation of flushed cheeks and perfect skin. I know, the novelty.

Manicures, pedicures, and the ever-rising bar of personal upkeep

Let's blame Jennifer Aniston for this one. True, the woman has suffered quite a bit in recent times, but my unswayable pursuit of the truth forces me to point out the telling synchronicity between Aniston's glossed-up appearance on TV and the mold-like sprouting of manicure, pedicure, eyebrow, and now Botox salons on corners around the country.

Oh sure, there have been plenty of actresses before who could combine that lucrative double act of looking accessibly normal yet obviously extremely well groomed. But none before did it as visibly as Aniston, because she was on one of the most successful and oft-repeated TV series in the history of the universe. Moreover, none before learned how to do this quite so publicly: a comparison between the almost scruffy Aniston of *Friends'* first series and her nigh-on unrecognizable appearance in the last provides an interesting lesson in just how much impact daily "treatments," an expensive hairstylist, and a personal yoga teacher can have on a woman's appearance and, by inevitable extension, professional success. And finally, she showed how, with just a bit of grooming, even a woman with naturally big hair and a face more cute than conventionally pretty might one day find herself up at the altar with Brad Pitt. That she then lost him to Angelina Jolie, a woman so well groomed that she managed to stave off frizzy hair when marching through Namibia, eight months pregnant and on the hunt for another orphan, merely proves the point. But since Jolie looks like she recently landed on earth from the planet Terrifying Cyber Babe Clone, while Aniston could easily be your friend from the office, the latter is more influential on women's behavior and belief in their own aesthetic potential.

Less than a decade ago, British women mocked what they saw as a purely and typically American obsession with this kind of grooming. My God, could you imagine? we'd marvel. All those nail salons on our cobbled British streets, taking the place of our noble eel-and-pie takeouts, our first edition Shakespeare bookstores, our sixteenth-century ye olde tea shoppes, or whatever other smug national stereotypes were wheeled out? Well, here we are, ten years on, veritably drowning in yoga centers, coffee "bars" (makes it sound a bit trendier, presumably, than "coffee shop," not to mention the Continental glamour of referring to your waitress as "a barista") and, yes, beauty treatment outlets. There are several downsides to this development. First, owing purely to their availability, it is increasingly an expectation for women to make use of such venues. Now a woman's preholiday preparations include spending a day going to her waxer, pedicurist, manicurist, eyebrow threader, hairdresser (for that crucial "sun and sea proctector" treatment), and fake tanner. The sensation one feels when trying to coordinate all of the above with that funny little thing known as "a job" is called a panicure. True, you could call it a medicure, but that sounds a bit too like medical insurance, although that, too, has a certain kind of aptness, as all this pressure combined with the required energy to schlep from treatment to treatment could send a strong lady into the ER.

It is one of those strange little facts that the fashion and beauty world spews in our faces now and then: the only people who have time to master all of the above are those who don't have to work. Yet few would be able to shell out the upwards of $60 necessary for each of the above (plus $200 for the hairdresser) without some kind of regular income. Thus, all this grooming malarkey has nothing to do with good style or even looking good; rather, it is simply another signifier, up there with vintage (see **Vintage**), of a life of indolent ease.

Masculinity, and the clothes that challenge it

It is a shame but not in the least bit surprising that fashion has accrued girly or gay associations. To claim that pride in one's appearance is solely and instinctively a feminine quality, women being such silly and shallow creatures, whereas men are thinking far too many big thoughts to have time to look in the mirror, is entirely in keeping with a lot of the gender-based nonsense that still, incredibly, gets spouted in the twenty-first century. It is also quite patently wrong, as anyone who has ever seen a portrait of pretty much any male member of the upper classes from the nineteenth century and before knows.

Whereas women are allowed to spend their Saturdays trying on dresses with their friends without anyone questioning their sexual preferences, men, understandably jealous, can only retaliate by clinging to the belief that taking an interest in one's appearance is a bit, you know, gay. In fact, a man would have to have serious doubts about the strength of his heterosexual convictions if he feared they might be pushed over to the other side by trying on a fine-weave sweater. This is what is known as irony.

And so men are forced to channel their perfectly human interest in fashion into more permissible vessels. Thus, they get pathetically excited over unbearably tedious things like ties, cuff links, and watches. Really, it's like seeing a dog having to make do with a table leg.

Even aside from fashion in general, there are some looks that are seen in particular as signs of an effeminate nature. Number one is wearing pink, but, really, if men would reclaim this (admittedly pretty objectionable) color, the world would be much improved, as pink would be divested of its girlish associations and therefore would not be used and abused in the manner it is now (see **Pink**). Second, tight T-shirts, but that's just because straight boys tend to get fat when they're over thirty so they have to think of some excuse for covering the belly. Next up, waistcoats, as sported by the lovely Simon Callow in *Four Weddings and a Funeral*, who was dressed by possibly the laziest wardrobe department this side of *The Matrix*. Again, this is foolish, as waistcoats are rather nifty, they cover up the belly, and, boys, you can have far more pattern fun here than you currently indulge yourselves in with your ties. With typical gaucheness, the once-camp pieces that the straights have reclaimed for themselves are, inevitably, the worst: cropped combats, gelled hair, designer jeans, and colorful button-down shirts (see **Party**

shirts: the fun-lovin' guy's staple). It's like watching a woman diet all day and then binge herself stupid on Häagen-Dazs when she gets home in the evening, stoically denying herself in one area only to then lose all self-control in the most misguided way possible. Boys, boys, boys! Stop kidding yourselves and let your inner sartorial soul fly. Get yourself some proper trousers—not ones that are apologetically baggy or try-hard skinny—just normal, good trousers; a nice top from a store like Club Monaco that suggests you might have a body under there somewhere and is in a not-too-garish color; a proper haircut; and some smart, plain shoes, such as decent brogues or sneakers that don't look like they were designed for astronauts. A facial wouldn't go amiss either, because pretending you don't have spots doesn't actually mean the rest of the world can't see them. It may not be the ever-so-manly pursuit of, I don't know, wrestling, but, honestly, you will find the results a lot more personally beneficial.

Mass market fashion, and the changing face thereof

It is now too simplistic to describe mass market fashion as disposable fast food compared to the indigestible haute cuisine of Fifth Avenue. Back in ye olde times all of, ooh, a decade ago, this might have been more apt, when the mass market was best described with reference to Bart Simpson's favorite cartoon, *Itchy & Scratchy*. But then European retailers such as H&M, Zara, and Topshop launched their plans for American domination and, lo, changed irrevocably the way America saw fashion.

Previously, American mass market fashion ran the style gamut of bland to dull. Basic white T-shirts. Ubiquitous-to-the-point-of-cliché khaki trousers. And although there is plenty to be said for useful basics, just because one does not have a bank account that can afford designer clothes does not mean that one is not interested in the aforementioned gear. An average annual salary does not a fashion-ignoramus make. Dammit, isn't America all about bettering oneself? Reaching beyond one's preordained boundaries? Maybe I expect too much from life, but somehow, wearing a pair of badly fitting, cotton-mix tapered jeans did not exactly make me feel like I was reaching for the stars. Moreover, because of this dichotomy between trendy-but-expensive high fashion and dull-but-cheap basics, the former, understandably, seemed irrelevantly remote to most of the general public. And then the European invasion. With their near-as-dammit versions of catwalk clothes, Zara, Topshop, and particularly H&M made what happened on the runways in Milan feel pertinent to people at shopping malls in Tulsa. Names like Chloé, Marc Jacobs, and Marni started being bandied about with blasé familiarity rather than reverence or cynicism. Instead of couture being seen as something purely for those at snotty charity dinners, one was afforded the indescribable joy of being asked whether one's dress was from Prada and being able to answer, "Zara, actually." And the cowardly American mass market had to catch up, as it could no longer hide behind the dull trousers it had been knocking out for decades, implying that customers couldn't expect more for their money, when that pesky Swedish superstore down the road was telling them that, in fact, they could. The Gap in particular, once a byword for the worst kind of American basics (three words: khaki, tapered, and khaki—or did I already mention that?), heavily overhauled itself for the twenty-first century, knocking out cute mini trench coats, pretty summer dresses, and cool shorts. Perhaps not entirely coincidentally, this very clever makeover was brought aboutt by Pina Ferlisi, whose previous job had been helping Marc Jacobs launch his ridiculously successful diffusion range, Marc by Marc Jacobs, which itself provided the style template for mass market stores around the world aiming to do good clothes (relatively) cheaply. Banana Republic, The Limited, and Express similarly all began to make clothes that showed a bit more sense of fun than one generally gets from a plain black T-shirt.

And the basics improved, too: jeans no longer cinched the high waist and ankle; T-shirts were cut properly to show that, actually, the wearer's armpit didn't bag down around his or her rib cage, and tops were cut sufficiently long so as to—oh novel concept!—meet the top of the waistband, so that the ol' muffin top was not on quite such general view. In other words, these were clothes that looked as though a smidgen of thought had been put into the design process, as opposed to just being knocked out blindly, expecting the customers to settle for what they got. In part, this shift was sparked by timing. Toward the mid- to late '90s, fashion was starting to get younger. Labels such as Chloé, Stella McCartney, Miu Miu, and, in particular, Marc by Marc Jacobs showed how to make young fashion look cool, by designing, respectively, pretty tunic dresses, slouchy sweaters, cute tweed outfits, and brightly colored basics.

Precisely because the clothes were so cheap, it now became acceptable to buy them and to pay attention to fashion in general. There is not a weekly celebrity magazine or daily newspaper that doesn't cover high fashion to some degree; when it was announced that the relatively little-known Phoebe Philo was resigning from Chloé, many of the broadsheets ran full-page articles. Thus, the mass market cleverly turned people's inherently prudent nature in on itself, making the majority, ironically, far more fashionably clued-in than ever before, because even though we weren't necessarily spending more money, it kept us up-to-date with what Chloé's new cuts were this season and whether quilting on accessories was in or out. Any twenty-something female worth her blond highlights was able to talk knowledgeably about Marni tunics and Luella handbags but—and this is key—in a savvy, non–Paris Hilton manner, because she knew that high expenditure was not an inherent sign of coolness.

The final triumph came when celebrities started to shop in mass market stores, as opposed to simply providing the template for the styles to be copied. There ain't nothing like seeing the blouse you picked up yesterday in Zara worn by a pop star being interviewed on the E! channel to make one realize that the gap between celebrities and mere mortals is really more of a stream than a gulf. And when it was announced that Kate Moss was to design a collection for Topshop, well, not even Trotsky could have conceived of a better sign that society had achieved some equilibrium.

Of course, the mass market is not perfect and, luckily for designers, never will be. What it is very good at is making fun clothes (as well as making clothes themselves fun). Party dresses, cute tops, jeans, summer frocks, bathing suits, costume jewelry, casual jackets, shorts, miniskirts—these should all be bought at mass market stores. What it is less good at, unsurprisingly, is making clothes that require a bit more time, resources, and skill than is available to your average Chinese sweatshop worker. Thus, good trousers, long-lasting winter coats, blouses, grown-up dresses, suits, and proper jackets are not so great in the $100-and-under outlets. Accessories, too, aren't necessarily the best investments at this level and are guaranteed to wheeze out and die long before those from a posher shop do. One could argue that, in fact, the mass market is to blame for the incredible rise in prices in the luxury fashion market in recent years, particularly in regard to handbags. Designers realized that the only way to stay ahead was to make things too complex for the upstart mass market to equal. Thus, handbags were soon laden with gold chains, big padlocks, quilted leather, and chain straps, none of which can be knocked off on the cheap without looking, well, cheap. Not only could the mass market not compete here but also designer prices inevitably had to rise, too, in order to maintain this level of complexity in their own wares. A similar thing began to happen with designer clothes and the suspicious rise in popularity of embellished garments on the catwalk. A dress covered in mirrored shards and Plexiglas pieces may dazzle when done well, but do it on the cheap and you look like a bathroom in a Moroccan B and B. People simply expect more from designer clothes these days, now that we know that, actually, it isn't that hard to make a camisole that actually fits or a summer dress splashed with a beautiful pattern.

And so the mass market ultimately made fashion both more and less accessible, and the world both more parsimonious and more profligate about clothes. And in an industry which can po-facedly tell customers that the fifties are very "now" and where underweight teenagers model clothes made for overfed bankers' wives, somehow that contradiction makes a mound o' sense.

Mittens, and the enduring appeal of pedophile-friendly chic

Did Mandy Moore ever wear mittens in a music video? If not, she should have. Just as Moore tends to play on the "little girl lost" image in her videos, all big-eyed, narrow-hipped, and generally half-undressed, so mittens evoke a kind of sweet, childlike helplessness that, apparently, some women think is a winner of a look.

Once you are over the age of eight there is just no excuse for mittens. Aside from the Imbruglia factor, they turn your hands into weird little paws so that you can't do important things like write text messages or attend to your Marlboro Light. This is what God gave you opposable thumbs for. Along with oversized buttons, frilled socks, Mary Janes, heart-shaped sunglasses, skirts with petticoats peeking out, and anything with a pom-pom, mittens are part of what can be referred to as, crudely if justly, pedo chic.

Pedo chic provides a salutary but aesthetically, morally, and intellectually upsetting lesson to us all about the dangers of taking youth veneration too far. While all women are trained from birth to think looking younger is better, the usual definition of younger, i.e., eighteen, seems to have somehow been mistranslated to four. It is the most extraordinary sight to see a grown woman in a cropped, swingy little jacket with a frilled collar, some sort of A-line pink skirt, and little buckle-my-shoe footwear, looking for all the world as if she were en route to her own christening.

Overgrown transvestite seems to be the style icon, and the effect is not to any woman's benefit. (And while we're here, why is it that when transvestites say they want to "dress as women," this tends to mean "cabaret bar owners" or "toddlers"? Never a simple LBD or a good pair of jeans or even just a brilliant H&M summer dress that everyone thinks you bought from Chloé—in other words, the best things about being a woman. Guys, you are seriously missing out.)

Pedo chic works in the same way as pink (see, yes, **Pink**) in that it is a very reassuring sartorial symbol that you are not to be taken at all seriously. After all, you're just a cutesy-wootsy little thing, a bit wacky maybe, but, you know, not in a scary way, who likes nothing better of an evening than to go home, lie on your cat-and-cuddly-toy-covered bed, and crank up the Dido.

Even if your appreciation of pedo chic is based purely on

aesthetics, ask yourself this: do you really want to hang around with someone who is attracted to a thirty-something dressed like a prepubescent? I mean, think of the potential for jealousy—no longer would you just have to keep an eye on him around other women at parties, but every time you passed a school playground during the day. Oh the stress! And stress, as you know, is just terribly aging.

Models

From Twiggy to Cindy to Kate to Gisele, one can trace the obsessions of each decade by looking at the models—respectively, stoned teenagers, aerobics, hard drugs, sex. For this reason, for all the fuss that newspapers make about the nefarious influence wielded by models on women's susceptible minds, models—possibly the most passive instruments of alleged control this side of Monica Lewinsky—are merely the reflection of the public's current insecurities and voyeuristic obsessions. Currently, judging from the number of underweight teenagers on the catwalks these days, today's fascination is—no, you'll never guess—thinness.

Models have always been, and probably always will be, thin. But there is no question that they seem to have become thinner every year since the mid-'90s. Everyone knows the old chestnut about how Western civilization venerates thinness simply because our meals and our bodies have become so supersized, and so, like moony-eyed teenagers with unrequited crushes, we all want what we can't have. Yet we seem to have entered a staring contest with thinness on this one, in that every year the definition of "thin" becomes literally narrower and not—it has to be said—just as it's defined by models but mainly by celebrities. Now that we are all so obsessed with thinness, a person can become famous merely for being thin—Nicole Richie springs nimbly if bonily to mind here—meaning that it's really celebrities who are getting thinner and models are having to keep up to stay within the public's increasingly warped perception of what is accepted as slim. But to watch a hollow-eyed model with thighs thinner than her ankles, her arms pathetically covered with soft down in the absence of any human fat to keep her warm, stumble mutely down a catwalk toward the aggressive mass of cameras is to see in action the phrase "taking an idea too far."

Newspapers get highly excited about the biannual Models Are Too Thin debate and how it affects women readers. It is an utterly reasonable, and probably long-overdue, argument. But, truth be told, with the exception of a celebrity court case, or maybe a royal family gaffe, nothing warms a news editor's heart more on a slow day than a story that can be illustrated with a photo of a pretty, thin woman. Funny how the word "hypocritical" seemed to float on the breeze there for a moment. Moreover, if some of the newspapers who have become particularly exercised on this subject were really so concerned about women's self-esteem, perhaps they could consider giving certain other stories—such as how working women are damaging their children, that a bit of cellulite on a famous woman is cause for repulsion, and how any woman over the age of thirty who isn't married and tied to a sink and a mewling infant is a selfish, stupid, probably celibate or, alternatively, sluttish tramp—a rest for, I don't know, a week maybe.

There is not so much a school as a mail-order course of

thought that says the reason models have to be so skinny is because all designers are gay men and their idea of physical perfection is the body of a teenage boy and that's whom they really want to, ahem, dress. We can swiftly dismiss this, and not just for its naked homophobia, and, yes, the word "naked" is being used advisedly. Briefly, any superstar designer with a million in the bank and a billion pairs of sunglasses to his name has, it's pretty fair to say, his pick of starstruck fashion-student teenage boys to play with; he doesn't need to console himself with a bloodless, flat-chested teenage girl from Detroit. If a designer wanted to design for men, there is a little industry out there that he probably would have considered as a career alternative. It's called "menswear."

In fact, designers claim that models need to be thin so as not to interrupt their "aesthetic," which is an impressively euphemistic way of saying that skinny people are easier to make clothes for, as you don't have to worry about boring things like proper tailoring, flattering cuts, or making space for bums and breasts. Instead, you can have fun with exciting things like peacock feathers on dresses and oversized puffa jackets trimmed with chinchilla fur.

Thinness requisite aside, the concept of models is a little odd in general. The point of the model is to insinuate that if we buy that dress/perfume/designer iPod case we, too, will look as good as the model in the advertisement. Maybe this does work on some kind of subconscious level, but you have to wonder about the qualities of a $1,600 handbag that itself needs to be accessorized with a $20,000-a-day supermodel in order to look hot. Wouldn't everyone be a lot more impressed with a shoe that made Rosie O'Donnell look like Christy Turlington instead of one that made Christy look like Christy?

Apparently not. Forty years on from Twiggy, centuries on from adoring portraits of society ladies and kings' mistresses, we all still love to look at photos of women prettier than we are. And this is the real issue. Designers use models for one reason: not to give us all eating disorders, not just for the sheer hilarious hell of it, not because they actually think we should look like them, but to sell clothes. If we weren't persuaded by a photo of a skinny woman spritzing a bit of perfume on her clavicles, they would have ditched that technique years ago. Equally, to blame models for causing eating disorders, as though their thinness is a deliberate personal attack, is even more stupid than shooting the messenger, as the messenger is the designer—you're actually just shooting the messenger's horse. The fashion industry doesn't give a fig what women look like—it's just interested in finding the body shape that hypnotizes customers into handing over their credit cards. So maybe we could just see models for what they are—walking, talking advertisements and feel, even, a twinge of pity while considering the physical exertions they suffer in the name of what is probably not a particularly fulfilling job.

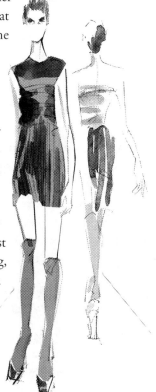

To say that models cause anorexia is about as incisive as saying advertisements for beer cause alcoholism. It is a mental illness. To make this connection between vanity, Kate Moss, and anorexia is yet another example of the media's infantilizing women (for it is, still, mainly women who suffer from anorexia, although certainly recorded cases of male sufferers are rising), implying they generally have too much time and too many copies of *Vogue* on their hands. But then, it's easier just to dump the blame on Anna Wintour than to ask why, in the twenty-first century, so many women still feel that the only way they can express inner unhappiness is through self-harm, I guess. This is not to let the fashion industry off the hook. It does intersect with eating disorders in that it validates the mind-set of the anorexic or bulimic. Thinness now really is as valued as they think it is. It's like the old horror movie cliché: you wake up and the nightmare is real. This may speed one's descent into illness and will almost certainly make it harder for one to recover, but it does not cause the illness.

Undoubtedly the fashion industry needs to expand its concept of female beauty, but it is just mirroring our own obsessions. Only when these change will there be models, and eventually celebrities, over 110 pounds, older than twenty-two, and maybe not almost always white. But let's not go too crazy here.

Money, and when to spend it

That fashion generally involves the expenditure of money is probably the most common criticism of it. Quite when the Western world came over all communist and decided that spending your own money on yourself was a sign of unmitigated evil is not entirely clear. Nor is it fully explained why buying a bag with a four-figure price tag is a sign of greater moral decrepitude than, say, making a terrible movie for $100 million (see **Vanity, and the joys thereof**), or why a $1,400 dress that lasts forever and makes you feel fabulous is less acceptable than a $1,400 holiday that is over in two weeks, leaves carbon footprints all over the planet, and is, if we're wholly honest, a bit of a pain in the neck.

Of course there is good fashion out there that doesn't cost half a month's salary. The all-new-and-improved mass market has confirmed that lots of designer stuff is a knee-slappingly hilarious waste of money. An $80 Stella McCartney–esque sweater dress from H&M looks remarkably similar to an $800 sweater dress from Stella McCartney. Designer pieces are usually (note that crucial hedging) better made, but badly finished seams are why God invented dry cleaners. And sometimes, when you pick up another poorly made designer blouse at Bloomingdale's and chuckle at the price, you do wonder if the designer just sits in his "atelier," flings a little ball onto his high-digit roulette table, giggles cocainishly when it lands on the $1,700, and puts it on the price tag. But none of this means you shouldn't occasionally buy something whose price makes your knees crumple in agony. People (i.e., your mother) will sigh and say things like, "Well, if you know you'll love it and wear it forever, then I guess . . ." but this isn't helpful. If people knew they were going to love something "forever," there would be no such thing as divorce lawyers. It probably does make sense to spend money on something that you will wear more than once, but, going by this logic, it is better to spend $300 on a designer T-shirt than $800 on a designer black-tie gown. In truth, the only factor that should dictate your buying something is how much you adore it right then.

Take away such distractions as a magazine article telling you that a bag is "essential this season," any photo you have seen of Kate Moss carrying or wearing said item, or any brain-fogging hangovers, boredom, or breakup pain, and ask yourself, Will the pleasure of owning this outweigh the guilt of paying for it? Will you actually be excited when you wake up tomorrow and see it in your wardrobe, or will it be like the morning after a bad one-night stand without the mitigating factor of being able to get it out of your flat before breakfast? If the answers are yes, yes, no, and if you can afford it without taking food out of your children's mouths, losing the roof over your head, and inadvertently funding some hideous Chinese sweatshop, then, what the hell, just buy it. Life is too short to spend it in bankruptcy, yes; but it is also too short to spend the next decade regretting not having bought that Cacharel dress which would have worked for every single party you have attended since.

People will often tell you that you shouldn't buy this season's It bag, dress, or whatever a celebrity has recently been photographed wearing because (a) you will be deemed to be a fashion victim, (b) everyone else will have it, too, and (c) it will be So Over by next season. These points are, if just, a little unfair to consumers, as they assume the only thing that could make someone desire something is pressure from the media. If your adoration overpowers the knowledge that lots of annoying people will buy it as well and that even more annoying people will sneer at it being "last season" next season (although surely everything is, literally, last season when we reach next season, but pedantry is a most unattractive quality), and you still don't care, then what the devil?

A few points of cau-
tion. Ask among your
trusted designer-buying
friends which labels can
be relied on for
decent qual-
ity. Next, ask
yourself hon-
estly whether
you will really be
able to use or wear it
more than three times. If the answer's no, head to the nearest
coffee house and do some solemn soul-searching about whether
you want to own a $3,000 dress that would ultimately cost you
$1,000 per wearing or if it will give you nausea every morning
when you open your closet, and, really, no woman should be
put off her Cheerios like that. Finally, think of a friend or even
a celebrity whose taste you admire and ask yourself what they
would do. This does not mean you should try to dress or look
like someone else, but rather that you should emulate their self-
restraint. Life can be pretty boring sometimes and a little
depressing, too. So everyone could stop beating themselves up
about spending money on their clothes and the world would
continue to spin. You're not eating small children, you're not
flogging WMDs, you're just buying a damn dress.

This is not to say you should come over all Ivana Trump and
forget that "designer" is a treat, not the norm. After all, like pea-
nut butter—or other substances with which some designers and
models are more *au fait* than nut-based spreads—designer pieces
are good only when used sparingly. If fashion is about self-

indulgence, the occasional guilt-free expenditure says someone knows she is worthy of the sporadic spoil; head-to-toe *Ab Fab*-ness says you accrue self-esteem only from having a screechingly camp, dead designer's name tag on the back of your skirt.

Moss, Kate, and how she ruined your wardrobe

Kate Moss raises many mind-teasing questions. Does she really think singing is a good career move? How did no one notice that her name should be cockney rhyming slang for "weight loss" until Lily Allen pointed it out? And why did she ditch the career-saving decision never to talk on camera in order to star in a mobile phone ad?

The most interesting one of all, though, regards her true calling. To whit, this young lady has not started a single fashion trend that has benefited womankind. This is not generally cause for ostracism but is a bit of a sticking point for someone so frequently described as a "trend setter."

Pirate boots, hot pants, waistcoats, pixie haircuts, expensive vintage dresses, furs, skinny jeans, high-waisted jeans—all started by Mossy—are harbingers of more aesthetic harm to the female populace than hair crimpers.

So perhaps the real question here is not one about Moss but rather—solemn dip of the head—about us. Because although most women have learned painful lessons from some if not all of the above, we persist in studiously following Moss's every wardrobe decision, certain she has found some heretofore unknown fashion trick that will turn us all into, well, her. The fact is that after several thousand years of getting dressed, there is very little in the way of clothing that remains unplumbed, hence the constant recycling of trends (see **Decade rehashing, and why designers live in the past**). What Moss does is find something that would look terrible on most people but looks quite good on her. Gather close, children, because here is an important lesson: that is why she is a model and you are not (see **Models**).

So while it is easy to understand why designers love her, it is less clear why so many women do, considering the damage she has wreaked upon their wardrobes, bank accounts, and dignity. Yet one could see this as cheering proof of women's self-esteem and optimism. Contrary to all the guff about models destroying women's self-confidence, the fact that so many women bought nasty suede boots with weird buckles in the belief that this would make them look like an underweight, photogenic twenty-something really does suggest they are not bothered by, almost certain, negative comparisons. And Kate, God bless her, keeps on proving this again and again as each trend she starts is more unflattering to women than the last, yet still we follow in her pixie-booted footprints. It's a darn clever strategy on her part to disprove all the media's whining about her being a bad example and the cause of eating disorders, because anorexia, you know, never existed until 1991. Bless you, Kate. Bless you and your high-waisted jeans.

Pantyhose, stockings, and the pleasures of a chastity belt

There are pantyhose ladies and there are stockings ladies, and the latter are simply wrong. Even leaving aside the silliness of their garment of choice, which we shall elaborate upon shortly, the criticisms they make of pantyhose are—now, let's see, how would Anna Wintour put this, ah yes—boneheaded. First, they claim that pantyhose is "unsexy." This accusation is predicated on the idea that sexiness is dependent on gynecological access, an idea that is desperate, overly graphic, and utterly, utterly ridiculous. Sexiness, wiser types have said for centuries, is all about suggestion, which really means, when it comes to clothes, ease of removal, and it's hard to think of many things easier to wiggle off than a pair of pantyhose. Stockings, on the other hand, have all these fiddly clips that twist up your underwear, and when the clips snap on inconvenient body parts, well, let's just say that an element of surprise does not always stoke the flame of passion.

Nor, while we're at it, do red marks around your thighs from where the stockings have been squeezing into you, whereas pantyhose, oh blessed contraption, make you look as smooth as a late-night DJ's voice. Yes, it may be the classic male fantasy to see a woman in stockings, but the key word there is "fantasy." At no point has any man ever lain back in bed and thought: "Oooh, you know what really gets the old motor going? Seeing a nice pair of thigh muffin-tops. Oh, baby!" And if he has, he's probably the psycho from *The Silence of the Lambs*, who throws women into pits and then grooms his yappy little dog. There's a lesson in there. Buried very deeply, admittedly.

Next, the nonsense about pantyhose being "unsanitary." Quite how anyone can maintain the argument that an extra layer of protection is less sanitary than exposure to all and sundry has never been made fully clear to the author. Moreover, having to fiddle about every time you need to go to the loo doesn't exactly sound like the most hygienic way to spend your day.

Finally, they say pantyhose is somehow "claustrophobic." Good God, woman, do you normally go commando? And you whine about pantyhose being unsanitary?

All women have felt the fear and, in some cases, the reality of walking around with their skirts tucked into the back of their knickers. Standing at the bus stop when your garter clip snaps, leaving your stocking to pool around your ankle, and then trying to refasten it without being arrested for lewd behavior while your fellow commuters snigger with undue pleasure, is pretty much just as humiliating. And unless Sharon Stone in *Basic Instinct* is your personal icon, you can't cross your legs or even just reach your arms above your head when wearing stockings with a short dress. Pantyhose renders high hems nigh-on modest, but always get it a size too big. This is not because you are fatter than you think but to allow extra length in the leg so that your gusset doesn't hang out from below your skirt like an incontinence diaper.

Even more tedious than stockings propaganda is the idea that bare legs are the sexiest of all. Flesh may be more seductive than material, but flesh riddled with goosebumps is not. Nor is a woman hobbled by frostbite or rendered mute by hypothermia most people's idea of sex on a stick. The nude look is dependent on a taxi or chauffeured-car lifestyle, as opposed to standing around and waiting for the night bus.

Of course, as George Orwell taught us, slightly paraphrased, whereas all pantyhose are created equal, some are more equal than others, and the ones that are the legwear equivalent of Napoleon the ruling pig are lovely thick wool or cashmere tights. Unlike silly sheer ones, these simply get on and do what tights are meant to do, namely, keep you warm and keep the world ignorant that you haven't shaved your legs since August. They make no apologies for being tights, as those awful flesh-colored ones do, which end up giving you an intriguing peg-leg look. They are also immensely more flattering than the black sheer ones that only ever looked good on the women on *L.A. Law* when they perched on their boss's desk and switched their skinny legs about. And lest we forget, these women wore blazers with shoulder pads and so are perhaps not to be trusted on matters of style.

While tights are brilliant and to be celebrated, let's not get too carried away with the revelry. Gray, brown, and black are the only acceptable colors—everything else is reserved for those who want to look like they've stepped out of Nintendo Land. Patterned tights were fun for about five minutes in 2002. Then one day we all woke up, collectively slapped our heads, and realized we were walking around with polka dots on our calves. Everyone sensible rightly chucked them in favor of plain or, at most, ribbed ones, which lengthen the leg and thus are very much for her pleasure, bada bing, and so on.

Fishnets, however, have lasted, and just when they seem to be dying out, they grab a last wheeze of oxygen around the office at Christmas-party season. At first there was something quite intriguing about their resurrection, in that it looked like women were reclaiming a garment heretofore freighted with negative associations. But the problem with fishnets is their aspiration for cartoonish sexiness, tricked off with a halfhearted attempt at irony. Irony, like "wit," may be occasionally acceptable in a personality but is rarely a good look. Oversized fishnets were a little more interesting, but you have to ask yourself if you want your calves to resemble the day's catch. They snag after one wearing, they don't keep you warm, and they leave crisscrossing red marks up your legs as though you've caught some tropical skin disease. A potential conversation starter, yes, but possibly not the party look every little girl dreams of pulling off one day.

Party dresses, and what yours say about you

When it comes to party dresses there is only one commandment: wear an outfit that makes you feel good. However, it often gets confused with a distantly related but very different rule: dress in what you think makes the opposite sex feel good. This tends to result in a yawning aesthetic gap between wishful thinking and impressive self-delusion. Hence the all-too-common sight of a winsomely girlish party dress on a woman definitely old enough to know better, looking more like the batty fairy godmother than Cinderella. Conversely, while it is all well and good to use a party to reveal your hidden sexual depths, the sight of a shy woman in a Lycra leopard-print dress gritting her teeth determinedly and sashaying in front of her quarry probably wouldn't have turned on Warren Beatty in his much vaunted heyday.

The real difficulty in finding a good party dress is that, with this outfit, more than any other, most people aspire to please simultaneously three groups with diverging requisites: the opposite sex, your friends, and you. Kate Moss, unsurprisingly, has mastered this feat with her penchant for shimmery (fun for her), long (respect from her girlfriends for going down such a maverick party-dress route), and body-clinging (hello, boys) party gowns. But then, she has had a bit of practice so don't feel too much of a comparative failure. On top of its practical difficulties no other outfit is more revealing about the wearer. On the flip side of youthful delusions and dubious aspirations to femme fatale status is "the lamb dressed as mutton": a young woman who prematurely embraces styles for the middle-aged matron. Sometimes they do this because they are preppy fools, and therefore we need not worry about them too much because wearing silk neck scarves and cable-knit sweaters seems to make them happy, seeing as they have been doing it all their lives. For women not from New York's Upper East Side or tony New England, it is often done out of shyness. Dressing like a middle-aged frump heads off the expectation that they will be the life of the party and allows them to scuttle home ASAP. It's the sartorial equivalent of self-deprecation. This is not just a shame but a vicious circle, because if there's anything that will put a damper on any potential party spirit it's some mumsy blouse, badly fitted jeans, and scruffy flats—a party outfit that positively screams crippling inner repression. As we've seen with the leopard-print Lycra, repressed feelings will only burst out in one inappropriately large gush, which will surely send the poor woman rushing back to her beige blouse. Ladies, ladies, there is a middle path! Even just a simple LBD with a bit of detailing around the neck, one bared shoulder, a gentle pouf to the skirt, or, if you're feeling particularly wild, a spot of beading will put you in a much better mood and not make you feel like you're the after-dinner entertainment at Club Med Cancún.

There are lots of "fun" party dresses out there, with ruffles (see **Ruffles: from French ingénue to Bozo the Clown**), patterns (see **Patterns—or test patterns?**) and velvet detailing (see **Velvet, and why it should be banned**). But as that ominous slew of parentheses suggests, these are fraught—fraught, I say—with danger. While each can work when treated with caution, designers too often abandon this, along with taste, practicality, and decency, at the sight of a party dress.

Worse is the broad interpretation of "fun" in fashion. A "fun" dress should be one that makes you look and feel witty and dazzling, rather than like an extra in the circus, possibly Chintzy the Clown. Of course, you don't want to just wear some boring black cocktail dress as if you were Barbara Bush swanning about at some tedious high-powered do with Henry Kissinger. But a compromise can be found between some nondescript shift and a bright pink satin affair decked with bows and sequins that might appeal to Fergie from the Black Eyed Peas.

It cannot be stressed too often—although heaven knows this book will try (see **Heels: the highs, the lows, and when fat is better than thin**)—how completely and utterly stupid it is to wear painful shoes to a party. Even if you're wearing a dress dipped in a magic potion guaranteed to make all who see you prostrate themselves at your feet, painful shoes will leave you miserable, grumpy, and boring. So dresses that can be worn with pretty flats are invaluable, and all the heel-philes out there will be surprised at how many such dresses are out there. With the exception of those just below the knee and mid-calf, most dresses can be worn with flats, with the hemline rising according only to your fondness for your legs. Although your legs may look less "toned" than they do in heels, this is not necessarily a bad thing, as in this instance "toned" is a euphemism for "throbbing with pain." And anyway, for all the sneering we do at their shallow depths, most men would rather spend an evening with a lady whose legs might not be hiked up to her armpits but is able to carry on a witty conversation than with a long-limbed goddess who spends the night sitting grouchily in the corner looking like she needs to switch to All-Bran.

Chunky, heeled boots are also useful if the thought of wearing flats at a party makes you inwardly, if misguidedly, recoil. These are great with tunic dresses, which have themselves been a recent boon to women. Essentially long T-shirts, these allow a lady—of any age, incidentally—to eat without annoying waistband strangulation, dance because they are amenably loose, and look good in a way that appeals to her friends, potential onlookers, and herself. They are loose, short, cool, and modest, four highly desirably party-dress qualities, three of which are in all-too-scarce supply.

A similar point can be made about keeping warm. Female party guests often assume that the more flesh they show, the sexier they are. Again, men find it far more attractive to see a woman in, say, a long-sleeved short dress and tights (an outfit that looks brilliant with, yes, flats) laughing and chatting and dancing all night than one in a spaghetti-strapped slip shivering miserably by the radiator and incapable of even saying "yes" when asked if she'd like to dance, as her lips have frozen together.

Other than the inadvisability of Cartland-esque pink, there are no rules in regard to colors and lengths of party dresses. It's all about what makes you feel at your most dazzling. Metallics are quite useful in providing the shimmer factor, without recourse to sequins, which can make you look like you're wearing an eight-year-old's art project. But be sure your metallics are slightly dulled, to head off any tinfoil jokes. The one exception to the anti-sequin rule is if the sequins are the same color as the fabric; they then can look surprisingly tasteful. They will, however, still fall off the dress, as sequins almost always do, meaning that, like Hansel and Gretel, you will leave a little trail behind you all evening, which might be quite useful should your friends lose you. Of course, black is the most useful just in terms of being able to wheel the old girl out the most often (and that refers to the dress, by the way, not you) without obnoxious people passing snide comments (and if they do, a brief reply is advised, one that involves the words "life," "get," and "a" in the appropriate order). Instead, party dresses are one of those rare purchases for which you don't—shouldn't, even—make a token effort to remember what is in this season; even fashion people know that this is one scenario in which looking good trumps looking trendy, hence Moss's long-term devotion to one style. You should also have some fun (again, I use that word with caution) with your party dress. This might mean wearing a heretofore untried style or what American TV psychotherapists call "stepping out of your comfort zone." Of course, you shouldn't step so far out that you become a social cripple (à la the shy girl in the leopard-print dress). But if you're generally a loose, let-it-all-hang-out kinda lady, at least try a structured cocktail dress or, if you're a floor-length gal, give a mini tunic dress a go. Neither of these is a particularly difficult style, and a party is probably the one place you can try out a new look without being on the receiving end of too many annoying comments, simply because everyone goes for a bit of self-reinvention at a party. Sometimes it's just nice to pretend you're someone else for the evening (in a mentally hinged way) or to take yourself out of your usual worries for a night, and it's ultimately cheaper, and definitely more attractive, to do this with a dress than it is with another partygoer favorite, drugs.

This is why it is not all that ridiculous (which doesn't mean that it isn't a little ridiculous) that so many women insist on buying a new dress for every party: if a party provides the opportunity for self-reinvention, then wearing a dress speckled with snakebite stains from that drinking competition at your best friend's thirtieth really isn't going to help you escape the memories of your sordid past.

Office parties are a whole other bag of chips. The problem with the office is that the outfit's goal is so different from that for your normal, garden-variety party—namely, to impress your friends and make every man in the room wish, to quote the wisdom of Kylie, that they could be so lucky. Of course, this latter goal may well, in fact, be your intention at the office party, inspired by a long-nurtured, hands-brushing-over-the-photocopier crush, but the reader is strongly counseled against pursuing this scenario. It can end in only one of two ways: either, one, a nasty breakup, resulting in daily bouts of crippling awkwardness and a custody fight over the office canteen or, two, marriage, which doesn't necessarily preclude the aforementioned.

So leaving that aside, your goal at an office party is to look nice, perhaps in something more interesting than the generic wrap dresses every other woman will be wearing—if only to show colleagues that you are far superior to them—but nothing so interesting that it will attract sarcastic comments all night from John in accounting or, more annoyingly, your boss. More pressingly, while you want to look nice, you would probably like to get through the evening without any drunken propositions, gropes, or eyeballs scuba diving into your cleavage. So think a nice plain dress, knee-length ideally, black almost certainly, but perhaps with a slash neck, bell sleeves, or maybe some detailing along the hem—something, anyway, to show a bit of style awareness (all bosses like to see that their employees are down wit' da yoof, and only in an office party is this proven via some pretty sleeve detail from Banana Republic). A trouser suit can also work as long as you leave before John gets too drunk and starts making lesbian jokes. Inwardly repeat the following mantra all night: "Friendly but aloof, friendly but aloof."

For weddings, there is no choice but to dress in something generic and just suck it up. A wedding is the bride's day, and any guest who turns up in some amazing Roland Mouret cocktail dress or whatever limited-edition Balenciaga slip that Kristin Scott Thomas was recently photographed wearing is being self-ish and stupid. Weddings are one of three occasions from which the photos are guaranteed to last forever (the other two being births and a really bad holiday). And as anyone who has ever seen photos from a 1970s wedding knows, nothing looks more comical to future generations than overly fashionable party clothes from times gone by. This doesn't mean you have to embrace the wedding guest cliché too enthusiastically; in fact, even though you're taking one day off from your lifetime mission of pushing fashion forward, you don't need to opt for the Pavlovian selection of a floral bias-cut skirt from Paul Smith, a pastel top from The Limited, and an Hermès silk scarf. Instead, something from the shift dress family, a sleeveless fitted top with a modest skirt, or well-cut light-colored trousers with a smart blouse and a hat that doesn't make you look like Kew Gardens on legs would work just fine, ensuring you will look the best in the photos, but in such a subtle way that no one can accuse you of trying to steal the bride's limelight. Ha ha.

Party shirts: the fun-lovin' guy's staple

God bless the man in the party shirt! Here is a heterosexual (and Party Shirt Man is *always* heterosexual) male who truly respects the power of fashion. In fact, lots of straight men hold fashion in more awe than do women, proven by the fact that they think sporting a pink shirt might be sufficient to alter their sexual orientation, or at least make people think they have (see **Masculinity, and the clothes that challenge it**). Women, however, judging by the annual return of "masculine tailoring," don't seem to harbor such qualms.

Et voilà, the party shirt, the favored weapon of a man who is probably not known for his wild and crazy ways but, oh, how he wishes he were. And so PSM believes that if he just slips on a certain Paul Smith button-down not so much patterned but mosaicked with some hideous design, he will undergo a Superman-like transformation and his party-animal nature will be revealed.

This in itself is rather sweet, but the real kicker is that PSM owns only one of these shirts. He has such faith in the shirt's efficacy that he doesn't imagine that its powers will diminish by overuse. Thus, the very same shirt comes out for every party, its fit perhaps altering slightly over the years as the wearer's girth expands, but, incredibly, its pattern never fades. It is the most remarkable reversal of most females' mentality, in that women believe one must never wear the same dress to multiple parties. Yet PSM knows that the powerful effects of the shirt compensate for the sneers.

Patterns—or test patterns?

Like curly hair and body weights of over 125 pounds, patterned clothes have been a victim of—deep breath, sonorous tone of voice—The Celebrity Culture in Which We Live. Oscar schmoscar, owing to the increasingly prevalent belief that a person's career can be destroyed by the quick snap of a paparazzi camera and the heartless placement of the photo in the fashion disaster section of a magazine, the most important achievement a celebrity can notch up is an ability to pick out clothes that will photograph well. This is why, for all the extra publicity they might bring, celebrities are ultimately very frustrating for a designer. With the occasional and salute-worthy exception of the likes of Sofia Coppola and—snore—Kate Moss, most celebrities aren't interested in looking fashionable; they're interested in looking good. Being fashionable is ostensibly about wearing a look that is different from what has long been the mainstream norm, and this determined, occasionally even blinkered, pursuit of novelty does not always photograph well. Some might argue that it's good for designers to have their more outré tendencies forcibly reined in by having to placate the celebrities. Yet it is a little pitiful to see a man who wiled away his boyhood dreaming about the indelible impact he would make on the fashion world making party dresses only suited for *InStyle*'s red carpet roundup.

One thing that rarely looks good on elite pages of celebrity magazines is a pattern. Patterns aren't slimming; they don't tend to make you look younger; they rarely even make you look taller: strike three! Yerrrrr outta there!

This is a real darn shame because a patterned garment can be a glorious thing. For a start, it's just dull wearing block colors day in, day out, no matter how flattering they might be to your complexion. Yet because celebrities are now so influential on designers and often on the way we dress, patterns have been sadly pushed to the back of the fashion queue.

Of course, some patterns are far superior to others: Fey, prim, whimsical floral patterns have been beaten into ignominy due to overuse at preppy weddings. Polka dots, which we have already discussed in this book and will probably do so again at some point, are problematic in their evocation of Minnie Mouse and their association with pedo chic. Horizontal stripes will make you resemble the Stay Puft Marshmallow Man, who terrorized the city of New York at the climax of *Ghostbusters*—and look how he ended up. Paisley makes you look like a walking Lava Lamp. There is no question that tartan is what is referred to in fashionspeak as "tricky" (i.e., pretty bloody hideous) and will generally make you look like you're moonlighting for the Scottish Tourist Board. But when done in relatively subtle and similar colors, such as extra-pale blues, greens, and yellows, as opposed to the traditional scarlet affair, it can be surprisingly bearable. Just don't wear it on a button-down shirt with a pair of jeans, unless you're going for a *Deliverance* kinda look today. Celia Birtwell's gorgeous line drawings are one of the rare patterns—indeed, possibly the only pattern—that looks as lovely on a person as it would hanging up on a wall. Liberty prints have kitsch appeal and so can be worn only in measured doses, at the risk of being mistaken for part of the set from a carefully preserved 1930s house. Marc by Marc Jacobs is fantastic for vaguely retro '70s patterns, which are nowhere near as hideous as that description would suggest; think instead of bold mini floral patterns, star prints, and other similar styles worn by the kids on *Sesame Street* back in its early years. Tellingly, the other womenswear labels that do patterns particularly well—Marni and Miu Miu—are very much labels that girls get and boys often don't (see **Get: fashion that girls do and boys don't**). While a patterned top is by no means as boy-offensive as an egg-shaped dress, it's not ideal, simply because it intrudes on a man's purpose. For men, a woman's clothes are there to make the woman look better when they are gazing at her. Patterns make for an unnecessary distraction. A woman, seeing as she's sporting the clothes all day, often wants to wear something that can maintain her interest for a couple of hours, hence the appeal of something with a little more to look at than a plain white blouse. It's a bit like wearable TV without the risk of accidentally finding yourself face-to-face with Paula Abdul.

This is not an insurmountable hurdle. For a start, you don't always need to dress for men. But you can also compromise, which, frankly, isn't such a bad idea when it comes to patterns. The first hard-and-fast—and rather obvious—rule is only one patterned garment at a time. This is why it is never advisable to buy a patterned coat. Even the most pattern-happy female might weary of wearing the same pattern every day. One also has to be in a certain mood—generally a good one—in order to carry off a pattern. Having to wear a polka-dot winter coat when you're hungover, recently dumped, on the verge of being sacked, and generally a bit annoyed with the world will not help your general outlook (see **Coats: stuck at the nexus between dull and stressful**).

Next, think about where the pattern sits on you. Patterns may serve as a distraction from your pretty face, but they definitely do not distract from your body. So if you'd rather people didn't stare at your hips and upper thighs, which suddenly seem to be looking two and a half times their normal size, don't wear patterns on the lower half of your body.

But the real disadvantage to patterns is their noticeability factor. Patterned clothes jump up and down in front of onlookers' faces shrieking, "Look at me! Look at me!" Plain ones are the shy, slightly mousy siblings who stand quietly in the corner. And while we could all do with stepping out of the corner now and again, there is something to be said for subtlety.

So you really love your new Marc by Marc sweater with the kitschy heart pattern, don't you? Well, by the end of the week, everyone else will know how much you love it, too, because it's harder to get away with wearing a particular patterned item more than two days in a row than it is a plain one—unless you want to be known as "that woman always wearing that heart-print sweater." Thus, you not only have to do the wash more often (nightmare) but also you have to keep some kind of mental timetable charting when you last wore that heart jumper, and that splodge-print top, and that beaded cardigan, and that Celia Birtwell dress, guaranteeing that you're leaving a respectable amount of time between each outing so that the neighbors don't begin to talk. And really, is that why God gave you a brain?

Pink

Women—kind of annoying, aren't they? All that sobbing into their chardonnay about men, counting the calories of carrot juice, and singing along to Chaka Khan with only a hairbrush and a mirror for special effects—pshaw! Oh, sorry, the spirit of a TV sitcom writer seems to have hijacked this book. After all, it's not like any of us really do any of the above. Well, not in public, anyway. One female stereotype that I will grant does seem to have some truth in it is a general fondness for pink. Obviously, this is all the fault of the parents with that pink-for-girls, blue-for-boys nonsense. But really, you'd think a thirty-year-old woman would have been able to progress beyond trying to recapture the color of her bassinet.

Pink accessories are cause for particular concern. "Don't fear!" they cry. "I may have money to buy my own handbags but, really, I'm just a sweet, unthreatening girl at heart, who wishes she could still play with her Apple Blossom My Little Pony!" For this reason, they are almost more grating than an outfit in head-to-toe pink, which might suggest a certain Glinda the Good Witch hang-up but at least is so ridiculous it can be swiftly dismissed. Relegating the pink to the accessories is some-how worse, because now there is not even the illusion of irony, just the pretense of subtlety coupled with a decided lack of shame. The difference between a long pink party dress and a pair of babyish pink shoes peeking out from beneath a pair of black trousers is like that between a fully signed-up creationist and someone who appears utterly normal until they let slip some reference to dinosaur bones being just an archaeologist's "conspiracy." Show me a woman in a pair of pink kitten heels and a pink beaded shawl and I'll show you a lady with James Blunt on secret repeat.

Plastic surgery, and how all those 1950s
B movies weren't so far off the mark

So it turns out the zombies really are taking over the planet: huge swaths of the population actually have been brainwashed into flinging themselves onto the tables of possibly questionable doctors in order to become members of some homogeneous, dehumanized tribe, and the human race has started to speak in strange, once-unimaginable tongues, with phrases such as "knee lifts" and "hand Botox" becoming part of everyday parlance in women's magazines and certain planetary areas. With every passing year the Western world falls ever more in thrall to this obsession. (Between 2005 and 2006 in Britain—scruffy, low-maintenance, stranger-to-the-blow-dry Britain—the number of people who had plastic surgery increased by a third; the value of Botox shares, meanwhile, went up by more than 50 percent.) My God, if plastic surgery hadn't come along, think of all the millions of people who would otherwise be in the unemployment line! Never mind the doctors—just consider all the hardworking men and women who make the apparently endless array of sensitive TV programs about plastic surgery with Emmy-deserving names like "The Bloodiest Plastic-Surgery Ops of All Time" and "When Good Celebrities Get Bad Noses."

The Fox network is particularly fond of this genre. Leaving aside the matter of whether you would actually turn to a TV network that, with apparently no attempt at irony, describes itself as "fair and balanced," despite employing such fair and balanced luminaries as Bill O'Reilly and Ann Coulter, for advice on how best to knife up your body, this really is a most extraordinary state of affairs. This network rather fancies itself, as it would happily tell you itself within five seconds of making your acquaintance, the protector of all-gathered-round-the-hearth family values. Yet here it is, counseling women on how best to proceed in this most modern, shallow self-obsession.

Just as those homogeneous chain coffee bars make every street in America look pretty much the same and offer nothing but fake coffee (Christmas-themed coffee—I mean, honestly), so these surgical procedures make everyone look the same and create nothing so much as fake humans, not fake youth. For proof, just look at a picture of Joan Rivers. Is your reaction (a) my gosh, look at that sexy lithe young teenager or (b) good God, the aliens have landed? And despite Rivers's openly admitting that this is due to plastic surgery—as opposed to proximity to a badly run nuclear power plant—she has failed to dissuade the increasing masses of people from signing up for a little bit of what she's having.

I am all for a woman doing something that makes her feel better about herself. If that bump on her nose has made her so self-conscious that she avoids turning to the left in public and wears distressing headwear to draw away the eye, by all means if she has the money and knows a good doctor, why shouldn't she get it ironed out? (Because it will be bloody painful, and there's no guarantee that it will really work but, hey, a lady can try.) And I have no truck with the theory that it is somehow "antifeminist" to have plastic surgery because it encourages a false perception of how women actually look. Honey, if your views of how a normal woman looks are so fragile that they can be dismantled by a glance at some plastic, airbrushed woman, then you are not smart enough to call yourself a feminist. Plus, it's a pointless argument: if words like "scalpels," "bloodied bone shavings," and "six weeks of looking like a victim of domestic abuse" don't dissuade the potential surgical customer, it seems unlikely that "not doin' it for the sisters" will.

The real problem with this astonishing escalation in plastic surgery is that the industry offers ever more procedures, giving customers complexes about parts of the body one heretofore rarely considered. No longer are we in the age of a simple nip and tuck or liposuction. Now every last crevice needs attending to. Hand Botox comes back to mind. Cheek implants follow quickly. And let us not forget ear touch-ups, of course, for those troublesome creases in your lobes. It is the rare plastic surgery clinic that will not mention these to you, and more.

And why shouldn't they? They need your money. It's like feigning shock that junk food companies dare to buy advertising time during children's TV shows. When else are they going to try to flog their oversweetened fruit juices or their breakfast cereals that are little more than sugar cubes in milk—during a midnight porn show? (Though, actually, that demographic probably represents the rest of their customer base.) This is called capitalism, my friends, in which everyone is out to make money. The only surprise is just how quickly the public rose to the industry's unenticing bait. If anyone wanted to make an argument that women are simple children, easily led, and in need of sheltering censorship, then this is it. True devotees of the form have come up with a rather ingenious rationale for this pursuit: they call it "taking care of or looking after oneself." As I said, ingenious, not only for the suggestion that fighting against nature is on a par with going on a yoga retreat but also for the idea that injecting oneself with general anesthetics and botulinum toxin A, as Botox is properly if not very temptingly known, is somehow tantamount to giving up sugar. Trudie she's-married-to-Sting Styler has become the self-elected poster girl for this dichotomy, apparently seeing no contradiction between her insistence on eating only organic food that has been fed on the tears of virgin angels and her regular appointments with her Botox doctor. But then, maybe the botulinum is organic, too—who are we to sneer? This is known as a Driving the Car to the Gym mentality. Quite why people would spend three and a half times more on organic food in order to duck all those scary carcinogenic pesticides only to proffer their faces to a toxin that was once considered a potential chemical weapon is just one of those funny mysteries life occasionally lobs our way.

This mentality is also to blame for the escalation in surgical procedures offered as gifts. Once, suggesting that someone should have their nose done would have been seen as a bit of an insult; now, it is becoming nigh commonplace for husbands and, increasingly, wives to give their partners treatments for those special anniversaries. "Happy birthday, honey, have some lipo." Awww, it's a Hallmark moment. And where the idea of giving a nose job to a sixteen-year-old was once seen as a weird fetish of batty wealth, best exemplified by Tori Spelling and her generous father, Aaron, it is now becoming increasingly common. But ladies and teenagers, be warned: remember that Aaron and Tori ended up with many a deathbed recrimination. So that goes to show—just because you have a perfect teenage nose doesn't mean you'll grow up into a perfectly happy adult. Funny, that.

Ladies, is this really what you spent all those years earning money for, studying for, working for: preventing your hands from aging? swapping numbers for Botox doctors? having needles stuck in your extremities in an attempt to look like a twenty-something when the rest of you offers proof to the contrary? And moreover, why should we continue the already too prevalent trend of women suffering such physical discomfort in the name of aesthetic "perfection" while most men occasionally saunter to the gym but in all other respects become the fat, hairy pigs nature intended us all to be in middle and older age? If there's one thing to embrace about leaving one's twenties and thirties, it is that one might finally achieve enough inner wisdom to let go of the self-loathing and bodily self-obsession that is the tax one pays for being young. To embrace the plastic surgery industry is to spend your life hating your body, railing against the unalterable rhythms of nature, spending ever increasing amounts of money, and enduring great pain in a vain (in all senses of the word) attempt to fight it.

Prada: the frumpy but fashionable

Prada styles itself as the label that's okay for intellectual feminists to like. You have to wonder how precarious a woman's self-image must be to be damaged by showing an interest in fashion, and it is on this kind of knife edge, poised between careful cerebralism and mocking artificiality, that Prada balances.

Prada's reputation as the acceptably intellectual label stems primarily from the designer Miuccia Prada. Rare is the profile of Mrs. Prada, as she is known, despite Prada actually being her maiden name, that does not make reference to her university degree and youthful dalliance with communism, as if they were proof of her unique cerebralism. As for the former, this carries the not inaccurate suggestion that everyone else in fashion is an uneducated cave dweller who thinks Chekhov is a pattern. In regard to the latter, some might question whether a move from communism to fashion design is more suggestive of fluid personal values rather than a show of deep intellect, but that belief seems to belong to the minority, judging from the tones of awe in which this biographical tidbit is constantly repeated. Particularly interesting is how this label has retained its tight grip on the cerebral despite being just as, if not more, celebrity- and logomania-dependent as any other Italian label, including Gucci and Versace.

For a start, its fashion line rose to mass prominence when Uma Thurman wore a lilac Prada dress to the Oscars in 1999 and looked, as Uma tends to do, quite nice. Next, the advertisement campaigns for its sister label Miu Miu almost invariably star a celebrity, such as Selma Blair or Lindsay Lohan, neither noted for the height of her brow. And finally, the whole Prada bag mania started only because Miuccia cleverly put the brand's label on the outside of those rather nasty little knapsacks the company knocked out in the '80s, thus making an item that looked like it should cost about $15 from Target into a full-on snob-value fashion accessory. You have to wonder how all that fits in with the ol' communist credo.

Ultimately, though, it's the clothes that give Prada its image of quirky intellectualism. Turbans, big fluffy neon-colored coats last seen on Carnaby Street in the '60s, frumpy and slightly awry tweed skirts, William Morris–print dresses, knitted leggings— all these have been featured on Prada's catwalks in recent years. You will occasionally see a simple, pretty dress or sexy jeweled top, but mainly Prada is a label that places oddness above conventional sex appeal. Although you might quibble over whether a woman has to dress like a sociology lecturer, circa 1977, in order to feel that she is dressing only for herself, there is something to be said for a label more interested in the woman wearing the clothes than in the man looking at them. That Mrs. Prada does this and is then lauded by her colleagues as being the great intellect in the midst, as opposed to a barking, hairy 1970s throwback, is proof that maybe the fashion industry isn't such a chauvinist beast after all.

Red carpet, and what we can learn from it

Not much, and certainly not much compared to how much coverage it gets these days. Aside from providing yet another excuse for the press to publish lots of photos of attractive famous people, the appeal of the red carpet is easy to grasp.

Contrary to what magazines and, more commonly, celebrity stylists make out, what a celebrity wears to a big event is not all that important. Björk is still trilling away despite the swan debacle, and Meryl Streep is still somehow lauded as a fairly respectable actress despite never wearing anything memorable to an awards ceremony. And they dared to give her an Oscar or two; I mean, I ask you.

The red carpet's real appeal comes from the insinuation that, here, we're getting a glimpse of the celeb off duty; insight into his or her real personality, even if that insight begins and ends at whether she is a full-length or knee-length kinda lady. In truth, of course, now that the red carpet gets so much attention and is seen as such a career maker and breaker, any real insight into a star's genuine personality has been destroyed as swiftly as Björk's swan dress probably was back in 2001.

Many people give great thanks to the red carpet—mainly celebrity stylists and those luckless fashion magazine assistants, whose job it is to compile "trends from the red carpet" picture spreads. It is now not so much an open secret as just plain open how much preparation goes into dressing for the red carpet and how little of it has to do with the celebrities themselves. Worse, with images of Björk's swan and Céline Dion's homemade backward tuxedo dancing through their minds, most celebrities understandably, if disappointingly, err on the side of blandness. So if anything can be learned from the red carpet, it's when in doubt, go for the beige, both in terms of dress color and movie choices (ref: Jennifer Aniston).

It is unwise to emulate a celebrity on a red carpet as his or her aim is to catch the eye of as many paparazzi as possible, which is not what most people should be after on a daily basis. Thus, famous men should not wear monochrome outfits—white shirts with white jackets, ditto for black—unless they want to look like, respectively, ice-cream vendors or hired assassins. Even worse are—ho, ho—inverted tuxedos. You know, the black shirt with the white bow tie (see **Classics with a twist**)—very 1990s. For women, red carpet dressing is just impractical, seeing as it generally involves full-length gowns (problematic on anything other than, indeed, a red carpet) and plunging fronts—both impossible and overly pornographic for anyone bigger than an A cup—and no accessories of any kind (proof, yet again, that celebrities occupy a different planetary dimension than the rest of us. Do they not have to lock their front doors in Hollywood? Where are their damn house keys?). But there are lessons to be gleaned. For one, if you decide to wear a backless dress you must apparently accept that, in exchange for all the attention it gets you, you'll have to spend the evening standing backward, turning your face around to make a minxy moue (ref: Renée Zellweger). It's an odd concept, this dress style, because although its sexiness factor seems to lie in its proof that you are not wearing a bra, surely this then means that you must be very flat-chested. While there is nothing at all wrong with being less than bountifully endowed, it does suggest that certain elements of the fashion industry's aesthetic preferences have now well and truly infected the celebrity world and beyond. If you decide to go for the high-slit style, you will have to lean back on one leg and stick your other leg through it to emphasize your daring style choice (ref: Liz Hurley). Again, not generally a winner in the practicality stakes or, in fact, anywhere off a red carpet, unless you want to spend your evening debating with a police officer about what constitutes indecent exposure. In fact, though, the blandness and predictable stereotypes thrown up by the red carpet have proffered some useful tips. Although I'm not counseling a full-on swan-sized break from the norm, it is always a pleasure to see a short cocktail dress in the midst of all those goddess-aspirants at the Oscars, even if the *InStyle* fashion assistant does stick a caption on it, dismissing it as "very off trend." Similarly, a nice bright color is a pleasure amid all the pastels and faded metallics. Ditto for the emergence of a simple flat Alaia ballet pump among all the beaded Jimmy Choos. Reese Witherspoon and

Sofia Coppola are the modern icons of all these techniques and prove that "quirky" need not be synonymous with "daffy." Rather, they show that it means "pleasingly and prettily original," and don't ever let anyone tell you otherwise, as it is commonly used as an insult against any woman who dares to speak or dress like she has an opinion. So the lesson from the red carpet is that looking a little different is a beautiful thing, and god bless the celebrities for selflessly proving this by going the opposite way. Only the beige go beige.

Ruffles: from French ingénue to Bozo the Clown

A tricky one, ruffles. A lot of women love them in the misguided belief they add a bit of "fashion" to a garment—"fashion" here defined as any detail, no matter how ugly, that is introduced to, as your camp uncle might say, "jazz up an outfit." Beading, tassels, and superfluous lace-ups also fall comfortably into this category.

Certainly, a bit of a ruffle is not the most offensive item a woman can have in her closet (slogan T-shirts avowing the wearer's attractiveness easily beat the comparatively harmless frill), and, in fact, some have been used to beneficial effect. Chanel, for example, is a label that has long mined the ruffle in its successful marketing of the French ingénue look to trust-fund kids and rich old ladies around the world. But note, in this case, that the tweeness, the girliness, and the general fussiness of the ruffle is actively sought in order to achieve Chanel's often cartoonish style. Your feelings toward this style pretty much depend on whether the Audrey Tautou film *Amélie* made you want to dance out of the cinema and hand out daisies to strangers on the street or run from the auditorium and rip off your own head in order to flush the ocean of vomit out of your body just that little bit faster. Ruffles are—in a very tenuous way, admittedly—like sugar: ration yourself to just the right amount and you're onto a sweet little winner; get carried away and you will gag on a saccharine mess. This tends to happen when ruffles are used superfluously, such as around collars, which will make you look like a clown, a medieval court jester, or Queen Elizabeth I, none of which is a good daily look. Instead, they need to be given a purpose, and if you think ruffles can't have a purpose, well then, you are underestimating the power of fashion, oh ye of little faith.

The most common breeding ground for ruffles is probably down the front of blouses, alongside the buttons. This actually isn't such a bad way to sneak them in and is a clever means of drawing attention to your bust in a faux modest, oops-have-you-noticed-my-well-shaped-bust-well-I-never-intended-that-to-happen way. But make sure the ruffles are narrow to avoid the clown factor, and just as blouses shouldn't generally be worn by anyone further along the alphabet than a C cup (see **Blouses: not so librarian now, are they?**), blouses with ruffles should not be favored by anyone over a B cup unless she wants to look like a walking heart-rate monitor gone askew.

A skirt or dress hemmed with a wide (narrow would be pointless, as people would not notice it) loose ruffle works in the same way as a puffball or A-line skirt in that it will make your legs look proportionally narrower without the pedo-chic quality of those two stylistic tricks (see **Mittens, and the enduring appeal of pedophile-friendly chic**).

Similarly, ruffled cuffs on blouses and dresses give one's hand a dainty ladylike look, even when you drag your cuff through a dish of hummus at a cocktail party and have to spend the rest of the evening with hands fringed by mulched chickpeas. Plus, when you wave them about you can pretend you're Byron, mid-opus, an all too rare side effect in the world of women's clothing.

And that is pretty much it. Anything else is just fashion chintz.

Sex and the City: what it gave us and what it didn't

With the glorious exception of *All in the Family*, no TV program has ever illustrated more truthfully human relations and modern malaise than *Sex and the City*. No, of course we don't all have that much sex, and of course we don't have that much money, but for God's sake, it's an American sitcom—did you expect "gritty realism"? And when it came to depicting fashion, it surpassed them all. Here were four women who lived alone and earned their own money. Yet, despite spending at least twenty minutes of every episode discussing where they were next going to get some, they never dressed for men. Yes, at least two but mainly one of them did dress like total sluts in body-clinging Ungaro (Samantha) and nude Gucci (Carrie), but judging from the contentment on their faces when they caught their reflections, this was more for themselves than for anyone else. Sartorial masturbation, if you will. In any case, for all the praise the show's stylist, Patricia Field, accumulated for her impressive makeover of Sarah Jessica Parker from aquiline-nosed B-lister to fashion doyenne, the fact is that most of the time Carrie looked really, really, really silly—to boys, that is. The girls, however, loved her. Let's see, there were the Chanel leggings, the de la Renta couture ball dress, the Juicy Couture playsuit, the giant corsages—these are not men-pleasing clothes. Heck, there was a whole episode based on Carrie refusing to throw out some revolting feathered Cavalli top, even though her boyfriend was threatening to dump her unless she made some closet room. Rather triumphantly, she kept both the top and the boyfriend. To be honest, purely from an aesthetic point of view, she probably should have ditched the sweater, but, hey, at least she was having fun. So for all the guff about the shockingly antifeminist nature of this show, it actually was anything but. It was about working women who loved their jobs, dressed for themselves in supernaturally bright colors, had more fun together than they did with any man, and lived vaguely surreal lives whose day-to-day plotlines had only the shadow of a semblance to reality. So unless "antifeminist" has somehow come to mean "occasionally sleeps with a man," it's hard to see what the problem is. Just look at the above checklist: this show was basically an extended, American version of a Pedro Almodóvar film.

What it didn't give us was much in between. In this world either you're a fashion obsessive and wear $1,200 dresses to lunch on Sundays (Carrie, Samantha, Charlotte) or you dress like a butch lesbian (Miranda). Nor did we get much on the downsides of fashion (feeling fat, feeling broke, feeling generally pissed off). But as I already said, this was a fantasy, and American, and a TV show, and Mike Leigh was presumably busy.

Its only real fault was the character of the *Vogue* editor played by Candice Bergen, who fulfilled many of the weary stereotypes we have come to expect from the film world about people who work in fashion (see **Films about fashion, and why they are all (mainly) rubbish**).

That aside, this show did more than any other—or movie, or magazine—to remind women that fashion is for them rather than for the schlubby guys that occasionally come into one's life. Mrs. Bueller, hats off.

Shorts, and why they're great

Your opinion of shorts will generally depend on two factors: how keen you are on getting out the legs and whether or not you lived through the '80s. If the answers to the above are, respectively, "very" and "yes, but I was too young to remember them," then you will almost certainly be more receptive to the style.

At some point in every woman's life she will have to ask herself that crucial question: is it all about the tits or the legs? In other words, would she do better focusing her sartorial efforts on showing off the top or the bottom half? For those who fly the flag for the latter option, shorts are the saving grace: they let you show off your legs without risk of flashing your underwear or, worse, tights' gusset, with the added benefit of extra warmth. However, those who were conscious during the '80s will possibly find it hard to return to a garment that caused them so much mental trauma when George Michael wore it two sizes too small. Even some youngsters ignorant of this noble lineage (truly, today's young have no sense of history) might be a little nervous about dressing like they're en route to a 1970s disco. For these cautious souls, the city shorts were invented.

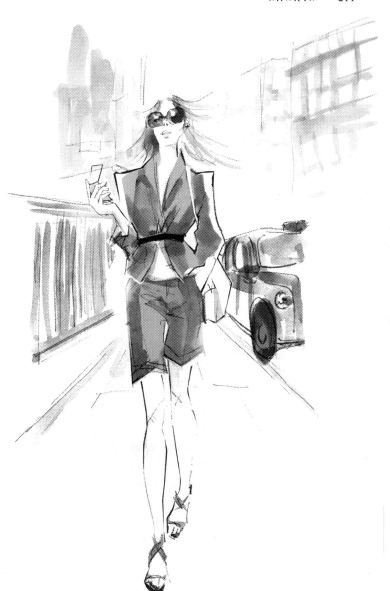

Be wary of any piece of clothing that is given a name that very deliberately evokes a mood or demographic. Think of all those designer bags that are, rather bizarrely, given names (Paddington, Roxy, etc., ad flipping nauseam); think Mary Janes; think Peter Pan collars; think kitten heels, for God's sake. Sometimes this is not a problem. Prom dresses, for example, are quite clearly based on dresses that did used to be worn to American high-school proms. But the term "city shorts" smacks strongly of retailers trying to give some kind of glamorous modern edge to something that actually looks, to the untrained eye, like a leftover from a local pantomime. "These shorts," the name audibly pleads, "are worn by the kind of glamorous people who stride the pavements with professionally blow-dried hair, their shades in place, making all sorts of exciting appointments via the BlackBerry while en route to lunch at Soho House with darling Charles and Nigella. Buy them and you'll get a bit of that action, too, you suburban slob."

All that said, city shorts are not actually a bad design. They are very comfortable, modest, and surprisingly fun to wear, in a novelty-value kind of way. But you do run the risk of being mistaken for one of the Munchkins, particularly if you are foolish enough to wear them with flats.

As for winter shorts—the recently resurrected trend for thick wool shorts worn over cashmere tights—this is again strongly dependent on how clearly you remember the '80s. It's a look that is jolly fun to wear but, to anyone over the age of thirty-five, will make you look like one of Debbie Gibson's backup singers. The triple layer of underwear, tights, and shorts can make you feel like you're wearing a chastity belt but, on the plus side, does keep you warm on cold winter nights, and for the leg-flashing lady, so used to winter overexposure, this is a rare and valuable sensation indeed.

Signature style

The concept of a signature style is, at first, quite appealing. In the fashion world, it carries intimations of a woman with such strongly defined aesthetic tastes that she is not to be swayed by the flotsam of trends passing in the seas of time, rather than, as cynics might sneer, a complete inability to conceive of more than one style of dress. You might think that the fashion world would be antipathetic to such madness, seeing as it spends a great deal of its time trying to convince the masses to adopt each passing trend. But, in a rather sweetly perverse way, fashion folk, and particularly fashion designers, are fascinated by people who pay no attention to their commands. Well, some people anyway, because it should be stressed at this point that a track suit worn three days in a row or last season's cropped jacket worn unaware that it's now passé does not count as a signature style. A true signature style has to be fashion aware, consciously cultivated, and either very expensive or very uncomfortable. This ensures that absolutely no one else will dress like you, which is quite crucial to grabbing the requisite attention.

The exception to this rule is a designer's suddenly being so inspired by a lady's signature style that he will base his next collection on her, marketing her look to the masses. This is definitely permissible, because if there's one thing better than being lauded for your personal style, it's being dubbed "a muse."

Dita von Teese (retro male fantasy) and Rachel Feinstein

(surreal '50s housewife) have inspired various designers' collections, perching contentedly in the shows' front rows while a bunch of underweight teenage models walked past wearing the same outfit as they were. This is an experience most women would describe as their vision of hell, but these ladies seemed to take it on the well-powdered chin. This muse thing does mean, of course, that when the designer has heartlessly ransacked our lady's wardrobe and moved on to the next woman—Wallis Simpson, maybe, or Louise Brooks, dead muses being so much less high maintenance than live ones—that "signature style" is going to look irredeemably last season. But like a young wench who has been ravished and then abandoned by the town's young bounder, she can console herself with memories of the time when she was the center of his focus, when Anna Wintour would nod to her at parties, and her name—oh glory days!—was in bold type on the party pages of glossy magazines in dentists' offices across the land. Now, though, she can only put that little pillbox hat on her head again, give her nose an extra pat of powder, and face the world with a fixed smile, letting them all murmur condescending admiration that she's still working that '50s look when the rest of us, obviously, have moved on to the '80s.

No matter what, though, once your signature style has been generally recognized and duly celebrated you can find gratification with the thought that at least you were once part of the noble pantheon of "style icons." Katharine Hepburn. Talitha Getty. Coco Chanel. Lauren Hutton. Audrey bloody Hepburn. Rare is the year that passes without one of these ladies being named as a designer's "inspiration" (see **Fashionspeak**) that season because of her "timeless iconic look."

This concept of a style icon is actually rather heartening because—unusually in fashion, or in the modern world in general, for that matter—one doesn't have to be young or even the least bit attractive to be one. You just need to have a signature style that is so strong and constant it basically works like a loud and very belligerent argument. Diana Vreeland, the nasally blessed fashion editor of *Harper's Bazaar* from 1937 to 1962 and then editor of American *Vogue* from 1963 to 1971, is the ultimate example of this. A self-described ugly woman with a voice never once described as melodic, she is still revered as a fashion icon thanks to her penchant for Chanel suits, oversized jewelry, and vampirically red lipstick and nail polish. She is the proof of fashion's occasionally democratic nature—a surprising result from one of the greatest snobs in fashion history, who once sniffed, "What do I think about the way most people dress? Most people are not something one thinks about."

For the rest of us mere mortals, there is a kind of watered-down signature style that most of us can and, indeed, do manage on a daily basis, called "personal style." This refers to the kind of clothes that you tend to wear in general: for example, if you are more of a jeans lady than a frock one, then jeans are your "personal style." Yes, most people would simply call this "having your own taste," but that doesn't sound quite as good. There are definite benefits to this "personal style" thing. For a start, it makes it very easy for your friends to buy you presents. It also saves shopping time, as a jeans lady would know never to bother going into Miu Miu, while the dress woman would rather carve out her eyeballs than bother with A.P.C.

On the downside, it does mean you will spend your life hearing people say, as they pick up something in a shop that is pretty much guaranteed to be hideously ugly, "That's so you." This is a very annoying way of saying, "That's so like something else that I think I have seen you wear before and would never, not in a million billion trillion years, ever consider wearing myself and nor would anyone else."

Moreover, your wardrobe also tends to be quite limited, and you'll realize one evening that while you might have an extensive collection of round-toed high heels, you have absolutely no strappy sandals, which are the only kind of footwear that will go with the dress you bought that afternoon for the party you're due at in forty-five minutes. This is quite annoying, too.

So look deep within your soul, ask yourself if, maybe, you're just hiding behind this personal style thing out of fear, neurosis, unconscious copying of your mother, or just downright laziness, and then get out there, girlfriend, and buy those strappy sandals. Cue triumphal end-of-credits music: *Chariots of Fire*, possibly.

Sizing: the nonexistent myth

When the subject of size comes up, it's hard not to come over a little bit atheist, because this is a god that empirically, emphatically, irrefutably does not exist. And yet billions of women bow down to its altar daily, basing their mood, day, and general sense of self on what this false god tells them that morning. Able to fit into the size 10 trousers today? Hurrah, life is sweet; you shall skip on down the street to the bus stop, patting small children on the head, and waving jauntily to the newsstand guy, as if you were starring in a Judy Garland musical. Can't even get them over your lower thighs? A cloud as dark as pitch swamps your horizon, you are filled with self-loathing, you slump miserably into that weird muumuu your great-aunt left you, and cancel that lunch with your best friend you'd been looking forward to all week because you have decided never to eat again for the rest of your life (until later that afternoon, when you eat two packets of cookies, because what's the point, you'll never be thin, may as well embrace the fatness, and at least Pepperidge Farm loves you, etc., and so on).

It is far easier to think of one's body shape as a 6, or whatever, than to bother bothering with the scales every morning, particularly since those numbers have somewhat lost their power to tyrannize now that every woman's magazine soothingly assures its readers that the scales "lie" because muscle weighs more than fat—a reassuring tenet, to be sure, when you see that dial moving upward, even if the most exercise you've done in a month is step up onto the scales.

Sizing also has a masochistically appealing suggestion of judgment, as though one were in the Olympics and watching the judges hold up their numbered placards: "Eight! Congratulations! You are the Russian of the competition!" "Sixteen! Loser! Back of the class with the Jamaican bobsled team!" That designers' sizes and stores' sizes differ compounds this sense: Armani and Zara might love you, but Paul Smith and Strawberry Stores just trample on your self-worth every time. Surely everyone knows a woman (possibly the one in the mirror's reflection) who rules out even looking in whole stores simply because of their stringent sizing. Some cynically witty mouths have wisecracked that a large part of the appeal of the Gap in Britain is that it uses

American size numbers, which are four lower than British ones. Thus, a size 12 is magically rendered into an 8 as soon as the customer walks under that blue and white sign, even if she did have two Snickers bars for lunch.

Yet this is precisely the point: sizes morph between shops and designers because there are no stipulations about the meaning of the measurements. Thus, just because a dress says you are size 10 does not mean you are a size 10 because a size 10 does not exist. Yet women who know that sizes are not immutable still quail at their power.

Designers have been able to use this fluidity of sizes to their advantage in different ways. On the one hand, you'd think it would be clever for a designer to make their sizes as big as possible, thereby appealing to the numerically sensitive and, unsurprisingly, quite a few designers have done just that. But on the other, just as fashion magazines seem to think that the classier they are, the skinnier the models inside should be, so some designers make their sizes as small as possible, suggesting that their customers are from the fashionably neurotic demographic. The mass market store has a slightly different issue. Unlike most designers, mass market stores have to bear in mind that a large majority of their customers are teenagers, and, thus, their sizes do have to be a little smaller, simply because they would otherwise have to put negative digits on some of their inside labels. Nonetheless, it does seem a bit tough on the adult mass market shopper, as it basically suggests that one has to pay higher prices in order to buy clothes with sizes that don't send you keening to the nearest trauma unit. So, although size numbers should not be seen as deeply affecting comments on your personal appearance, they should, nonetheless, be taken pretty personally.

Because if size numbers define the store's self-image, then a store whose sizes seem angrily unwelcoming is a store that is basically saying it doesn't want you as a customer. And you should respond in kind with a spin on your heel, your wallet remaining tucked inside your whatever-sized jeans.

Sunglasses, the meaning of

Funnily enough, there once was a time when sunglasses were merely glasses to be worn in the—ooh, what was it? What's the word we're looking for here? Oh yes—sun. Yet these little darkened spectacles are a true testament to the strength of sartorial semantics, the (deep, booming voice) power of fashion, and (slightly quieter voice) the intriguing mentality of those who work in it. During the course of the twentieth century, sunglasses became the symbol of, pretty much in this order, the rich, the famous, the cool, and the psychotic. In regard to the first, this was because in the pre-easyJet era only rich people could afford to jet off to Capri with darling Miffy, Biffy, and Squiffy for the summer to hang about on Jiffy's yacht, the *Tiffy*.

Then the famous got onto this shades thing, ostensibly to preserve their much-vaunted "privacy," although now that sunglasses are synonymous with celebrity there are some folk who would probably be unrecognizable without them such as Elle "aviator" Macpherson and Nicole "owl" Richie.

No matter, once they became signifiers for wealth and fame, sunglasses inevitably became symbols of coolness, seeing as these two states of being are the pinnacle of our collective life ambition. With unexpected conservatism on the film industry's part, these outward shows of cool bad-boy behavior became easy wardrobe shorthand for baddies, usually trying to kill George Clooney. But they are also as much of a cliché for people who work in fashion as Marlboro Lights. As most fashion people channel their tendencies to psychosis into compulsive shoe shopping and talking in non sequiturs ("Eighties! Essential!"), it would seem we're back to the first three meanings. There are several possible explanations for what's going on here. First, as we've already established, because the fashion industry is, at heart, a big business about playing dress-up, it has so stunted the emotional maturity of all those who work in it that they, like teenagers, still believe that refusing to make eye contact makes you the coolest kid on the playground. Similarly, they cling to the associations of wealth and fame, both inevitably venerated in their industry, as it is primarily those two demographics who are able to afford their clothes.

Next, that it makes them look ever so jet-sety, like they have to fly at a moment's notice to Jamaica for that shoot with Natalia before meeting up with J.Lo in Beverly Hills, never mind that air travel has long since lost its associations with exclusivity or glamour.

And giving a brief nod to the psychotic factor, there is no denying that hiding one's eyes makes onlookers uneasy. This is very good. Although fashion is ostensibly about the pursuit of beauty, it does venerate certain looks not considered desirable in the outside world. Frailty comes first to mind, but scariness is definitely up there. This is partly to keep the outsiders out, by making fashion look more complicated than it arguably actually is: if it were (blatantly) just about pretty dresses, why then, anyone would think (realize) they could do it. But cultivating hostility is also a career move. Whereas big city bankers might steal one another's clients and go on competitive drinking sprees in overpriced clubs, people in the fashion industry face down up-and-coming rivals by making themselves look as fearsome as possible—well, as fearsome as you can in a ladylike Chanel suit.

Sunglasses are also very useful for covering dark circles if one has been out a little too late with Kate and Lindsay and, like, everyone important at Le Baron in Paris doing—oh God, you couldn't even imagine what they were doing. Better still, sunglasses are brilliant at suggesting that this is what you were doing even if, in fact, you just stayed up too late in your hotel room watching *Larry King Live* on CNN. Thus, they become meta-suggestive. And you thought fashion was a shallow, single-layered affair.

Similarly, sunglasses are very good at covering eyes purpled by recent cosmetic treatments and so suggest that you've recently had something "done"—this now being something to vaunt, as it proves your dedication to the cause.

Finally, they mean you never run the risk of squinting, which, you know, causes crow's-feet. And so, to sum up, they make you look cool, they make you look rich, they get you attention because people think you might be famous, and they might possibly stop wrinkles—frankly, it's a wonder the fashion world hasn't put them up for sainthood.

As for what you do with them, this, too, is fraught with vital semiotic signs that one must learn in order to avoid Fashion Death. Unless you are a yah-yah-ing, white-jeans-wearing, honey-tressed prepster, they must never be worn on top of your head. This conveys two messages: first, not only that you wish you were an Upper East Side preppy queen who could wear a headband in peace without fear of mockery but also that you are a coward, as you refuse to accept this truth and are opting out with a weak headband compromise (see **Hair accessories: gimmicks for reluctant adults**) or, second, that you think you are so famous that you need your specs at just a moment's notice in case a member of the—ewwww!—general public dares to invade your personal force field. So keep them on at all times, except when you go inside, unless you are in a manufactured-boy-band video, in which case they serve to try to convince fans that you are actually Quite Hard. When you must, tragically, remove them, stick them in your handbag: folding them up and sticking them in your front pocket makes you look simultaneously like your dad on holiday and the leader of a minor principality, two images one would not have thought possible to evoke at the same time, but such is the power of sunglasses.

The most gripping development in sunglass style in recent years has been the rise of the oversized sunglasses. This trend was started by the celebrity stylist Rachel Zoe, the woman who single-handedly made people think 1970s caftans were cool and Nicole Richie was glamorous, and somehow, even more impressively, combined the two. The genius of oversized sunglasses is that they carry intimations of old-school diva glamour (read: you can behave like a total bitch but people will forgive you because you look so fabulous); they have vintage store associations even if they are now so popular that most modern designers make them; and they make your face look so small as to appear—reeee-sult!—malnourished. With such obvious attractions they have become the inevitable prop of every aspiring starlet and wannabe celebrity. Certainly, larger glasses are more flattering, but the trend for ones so big that they all but make it impossible to eat (and again, reeeesult!) is rather akin to the theory that thin is in, now developing into a situation where teenage models are dropping dead from heart failure. In other words, it's an idea taken a little bit beyond its originally intended meaning.

Aviators are for someone either whose heyday was in the '80s—hence their popularity among aging models and socialites—or who has an impermeable, and possibly subconscious, veneration of Tom Cruise, the early years, i.e., the midlife crisis man, and middle-aged gay men.

Colored and decorated frames are just great for those who willingly describe themselves as "a bit wacky." They are also fabulous for squeezing on some extra logos or Pucci swirls, should you feel that your Balenciaga Lariat bag isn't packing enough bling that day. This is perhaps the only instance in which these two demographics—the goofily tacky and the logo'd-up St. Tropézienne wannabe—overlap.

Impermeably black ones are for spies, bodyguards, celebrities, and fashion journalists. The first two use them to not be noticed and the other two use them for precisely the opposite reason. In this sense, black sunglasses are both an ambidextrous and a bisexual accessory.

As for mirrored shades, well, these are just creepy. There is something so deeply weird about talking to someone and seeing only your own self looking back at you, as though the person beneath is a soulless alien life-form. And considering they spent their own good money to achieve that effect, they may well be.

Colored sunglasses were once the symbol of an eco-aware pop star with aspirations to maverick status, despite being in the most mainstream band this side of Genesis. But then aging former hippies started wearing them, and now no one knows what the hell they mean, except maybe "middle-aged liberal who still thinks they're a bit of a wild card." Rock on!

Thin knits

Thin knits, baby! That's where it's happening these days! Eagle-eyed readers might espy the inherent contradiction in this concept, but first to its advantages. Ladies—and this style is one primarily for the ladies—like to be warm. But many don't want to disguise their charms wholesale. Even those who don't fancy risking hypothermia for the sake of heading out in a miniskirt mid-January generally don't want to resemble David Starsky, he of *Starsky & Hutch* fame, burrowing beneath a giant cardigan. Hence the thin knit, which gives coverage but not in great quantities. Yes, it is a bit sexier to be able to glance at just that hint of skin beneath an otherwise innocuous long-sleeved top, and, yes, thin-knit tops have been a boon for the layering (see, yes, **Layering, the whats and the hows of**) trend. But as knits are supposed to keep you warm and the adjective here suggests they won't do the job brilliantly, you'll need to buy and then wear at least three at a time, if only to keep from expiring of hypothermia. Sometimes, you really have to give the fashion industry credit for the ways they find to get people to hand over more money.

Not that the fashion world now denigrates the chunky knit,

of course, as seen in the cable-knit oversized sweaters by Stella McCartney and Chloé that are woollier than the whole of Wales. These (the sweaters, not Wales) have lovely connotations along the lines of snuggling down with one's boyfriend (boyfriends being much cooler than husbands, of course) in front of a big open fire in one's enormous but, you know, cool country pile in Shropshire or perhaps chalet somewhere in France. So, to recap, thin knits—good, in a flash the flesh modestly and frostbitten way; chunky knits—good, and warm, in a suitably aristocratic setting. Isn't it nice how fashion can see the positives in everything? Let the cash tills ring in the financial new year!

Toes, and what the shape says about you

Not your own actual toes, of course. Except if your foot is squared off, in which case you are, as all readers of Roald Dahl know, a witch, and you might want to bear that in mind, just for your own self-knowledge.

Dahl was, of course, quite right: squared-off feet suggest an inhuman nature. Yet while the witches endure terrible foot cramps attempting to disguise this physical deficit, some women today spend actual money on the reverse, buying shoes with squared-off toes. It really is the oddest thing. Look down at your little squared feet and ask yourself, What is it about this look that so appealed to me? There are many times one might suffer the inevitable lifetime of limping for the sake of painful footwear (see **Heels: the highs, the lows, and when fat is better than thin**), but going for a witchishly squared foot is not a reasonable motive. And stop that nonsense about their being "so much more comfortable." Any shoe that does not follow the actual shape of your foot is not benefiting you in the slightest.

I fully concede that pointy-toed shoes are just as unacceptable as their dumpy, square counterparts, and maybe even more so because the wearer generally has adjectives of the "sexy," "vampish," "Linda Fiorentino" variety running through her mind, when in fact they simply look mean. And let's not even get into the theory about pointed shoes being "leg lengthening": anyone who mistakes an elongated, pointed shoe tip for a long, lean thigh is someone whose limited intelligence disqualifies them from this discussion.

Both the squared and pointed toe work on the odd principle that your foot has a shape that everyone knows it doesn't. Yes, sometimes fashion does encourage body reshaping (padded bras, control-top pantyhose, corset-style tops), but this is generally because onlookers could potentially be fooled into thinking that the wearer has, respectively, globular breasts, a flattened stomach, and an hourglass figure. No one, surely, would look at a squared or pointed shoe and think it's the actual shape of the foot inside, nor, one can only presume, would the wearer want them to do so. Yet while the similarly bizarre and semiotically incomprehensible shoulder pads have, happily, long ago been relegated to an embarrassing joke, we hang on to this oddly shaped footwear.

Of course, to take this toe argument much further would be to suggest a diagonally shaped shoe, that being the shape of your foot and all, and that is probably too much of a leap as yet for the timorous pointed- and squared-toe masses.

The obvious compromise is the rounded toe. It is perfectly

pretty in an innocuous kind of way, it suits every shoe style and—and listen up, squarish diehards—it is comfortable. Now, the problem with the rounded toe is that, as proven by the plethora of upsetting ballet pumps (see **Ballet pumps: twee versus comfort**), it is surprisingly hard to do well. It has to look delicate, ladylike, yet not too exaggeratedly Minnie Mouse. The ideal shape is like that of the top of a slightly askew egg, with the high, rounded tip to one side and fanning downward. Marc Jacobs and Chloé have perfected the style, and some valued members of the mass market have learned their curving lessons. It can look a little too girlish, but this is generally the fault of the shoe as opposed to the toe, so if you don't want to look like you work at Walt Disney World, don't buy red polka-dotted high-heeled mary janes. A motto, perhaps, some women should have embroidered on the outside of their wallets.

Still, both the pointed and the rounded toe are preferable to the open toe and even to its cheat, the peep toe, simply because they are lower maintenance. There is a rather sweet theory that open-toed shoes are sexier than their closed counterparts, and this probably is true even if, seeing as the foot is not widely regarded as the sexiest part of a woman's anatomy, it does suggest that we haven't moved too far from the Victorian days of yore, when piano legs were allegedly considered quite the hubbest of hubba. Certainly the open-toed strappy shoe is a remarkably useful piece of footwear, because, thanks to its near invisibility, it can be worn with pretty much any garment in your closet. However, a woman who wears open-toed shoes is a woman who has time and patience in her life for weekly pedicures, nightly foot moisturizing, and a social life that tends to involve sitting decorously in glamorous bars in Ibiza with P. Diddy and Cameron Diaz as opposed to, say, waiting for the night bus at 3 A.M. in January.

The peep toe is, deceptively, just as demanding. Only one toe tends to be visible, but for that very reason you'd better make sure that toe is up to scratch because all attention will be on it. The peep toe has associations with 1950s starlets, burlesque dancers, and rather fabulously insouciant Frenchwomen strolling down the piers in Saint-Tropez. But one should never look for style guidance from a Frenchwoman; it would be like hoping to pick up mental arithmetic tips from Stephen Hawking—some people are just made from a different, more instinctively rigorous model than the rest of the human species and, for a Frenchwoman, a weekly pedicure is probably up there with monthly dog grooming in terms of obviously essential appointments. In regard to burlesque dancers, they presumably have bugger all else to do with their daytime hours other than schlep on down to the local nail salon while mentally deciding on which boa-and-corset combo to wear that night. And as for 1950s actresses, well, maybe there wasn't that much to do in the '50s other than get your nails done, seeing as cable TV hadn't yet been invented.

Trench coats

Trench coats, like the pencil skirt, little black dress, and "a proper handbag," is one of those items fashion magazines always say one simply has to own as part of one's grown-up, basic wardrobe, but actually it just makes you feel like you're trying to pretend you're in some terrible French film homage. At least

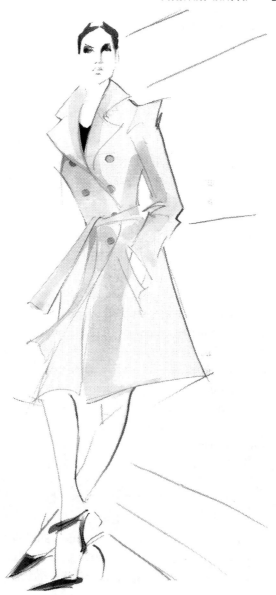

the pencil skirt et al. have rather glamorous precedents—
respectively, Deneuve, Hepburn, and Birkin—whereas few have
aspired to look like a detective with an *'Allo, 'Allo* accent. This
veneration of the trench coat is an interesting example of the law
of Dick Clark: if something simply hangs around for long
enough, it will eventually be applauded as "a classic." But the
fact is, like the pencil skirt, the trench coat doesn't actually suit
many women. It's a coat—but not very warm; it's for out-
door wear—but shows every speck of dirt; it's similar in color to
many women's skin—which just makes them look jaundiced.
And yet, and yet, on it lingers, haunting the pages of fashion
magazines like an old smell of cabbage in a dead relative's
apartment.

Admittedly, the trench coat can look quite chic on some
women. Kate Moss comes to mind; glamorous Frenchwomen
follow on her heels. But the former would look decent in a dress
made of cellophane, which, in fact, she really did wear once.
And the latter are foreign, so we just accept their peccadilloes.
But this is the truth of trenches: like all clothing, they suit some
people and not others. Amazing, *n'est-ce pas?* So don't be fooled
by this classic or, worse, "staple" moniker. A magazine that
describes a trench coat as a classic is almost certainly a magazine
gunning for that Burberry advertising account.

Vanity, and the joys thereof

When people knock fashion, their most common criticism is
that it's a vain, self-obsessed pursuit. But it's never been made
wholly clear why fashion is denigrated as shallow while cinema
or art or theater is lauded as spiritually enriching. These aestheti-

cally based industries also involve huge sums of money, attract appallingly egotistical people, and tend to exclude anyone below the middle class. Yet if you spend an evening watching some snotty folk snot about on a snotty stage, you are lauded for your cultural pursuits, whereas if you while away a harmless afternoon admiring some pretty dresses in a shop, you are irredeemably self-indulgent. Retaliate with this argument and you will be accused of being "facetious." Being a fashion airhead, I'm unsure of the exact definition of this word, but I suspect it means "annoyingly right." As for the argument that fashion is a hideous waste of hilarious amounts of money, my God, have you seen how much paintings go for these days? A Klimt for $73 million, wasn't it? Or have you checked out Tom Cruise's $100 million salary for the coma-inducing *War of the Worlds*?

Let's not get into the hoary is-it-art-or-is-it-fashion debate, mainly because it's boring, but also because it's a bit of a red herring in that it suggests that fashion has to pretend to be Monet in order to be tolerated. Fashion produces no more personal dissatisfaction than watching Cameron Diaz on-screen, is no less prone to whims and trends than the art world, and is usually a lot more fun than seeing *Hamlet* for the seventy-second time.

The fact is, feeling pride in your appearance gives you happiness and self-confidence. I concede that at times this does cross over into its opposite, with women laboring under a lifetime curse of self-hatred and physical contortion, and this is very wrong. But it seems similarly antifemale to insist that in order to be a true feminist one is not allowed to have any vanity. This is just a breath away from the old antifeminist stereotype about hairy armpits and burlap trousers—a stereotype that has led to a current generation of girls loath to describe themselves as feminists in the belief that this makes them sound like they're in favor of body hair instead of equal pay.

Patriarchal society or not, everyone likes to look good. Heck, even Barbara Bush gets out the lipstick on a daily basis, and, as that example proves, this is not just about looking good for the boys—it's about looking in the mirror and having a little smile.

Here, one suspects, lies the potential nub of the antifashion prejudice. Good God, women doing something just for themselves? Spending their own money? Women making themselves feel good about themselves rather than martyrishly chaining themselves to the sink and raising some cigar chomper's children while he's off shagging his administrative assistant? An industry dominated by—oh vision of burning hell!—women? Dear God, cover your eyes, think of the children!

I concede that it is difficult to decide whether something makes you feel better because you genuinely like it or because you are conforming to society's expectations. But perhaps we could all give one another credit for being able to figure that one out for ourselves. And look at it this way: it is a proven fact that you are more likely to get a job if you dress nicely. Object to the superficiality of this world all you like, but the truth is that the more women there are who look decent and feel self-confident, the more women there will be in good jobs so we can take over the world. And seeing as Germaine Greer is now busy discussing the joys of the Rabbit vibrator, I'd say *Vogue* is probably a better option these days than *The Female Eunuch*.

Velvet, and why it should be banned

The problem with velvet is not how it looks (although that certainly is problematic) but what it represents. This is a fabric intrinsically associated with two subjects particularly prone to clichés: namely, elderly women and festive fashion. Seeing as the queen provides the link to this Venn diagram, and, in fact, has long been partial to a bit of velvet, we may as well blame her.

To the older women first. With the exception, perhaps, of women who play the harp or sing in medieval music groups, there is not a female alive under the age of sixty who ever considers buying a velvet dress or, God save us, velvet trousers, except in very specific circumstances, and we shall return to those in a bit. (And if there is, there shouldn't be. This is a fashion book, okay? We deal in how the world ought to be.) Velvet is a fabric best reserved for a country club Christmas luncheon. Yet somehow it has become ingrained in women's minds that this profoundly and garishly ugly material is what they should wear as they enter their seventh decade. It is clumsily heavy yet unflatteringly clingy, and the way it changes color tone when the pile is rubbed the wrong way makes it look like it's covered with dribble stains.

Now, if older women actually liked it, that would be fine—odd, but fine. Yet the uniformity of the point at which they start wearing it suggests that wearing velvet, like suddenly becoming partial to doilies or fancying Regis Philbin, is something they do because they think they should. The fact that clothing manufacturers seem to think so, too, and therefore get rid of all their velvet offcuts by unloading them on the—snigger—blue-hairs may have even more to do with it. But if there's one time in life when you shouldn't be embracing clichés it's when you get older. C'mon, you're still alive and kicking (albeit perhaps not as high as you used to). Just because Talbots says you have to start dressing the way you remember your granny did doesn't mean that you do. There's enough ageism out there without you conforming to its worst diktats. Get on down to Zara, ma'am, find yourself a nice sharp jacket and blouse, and wear them with your favorite trousers for walking the poodles.

Festive dressing is also a victim of enforced sartorial stereotypes, as if sitting around for seventy-two hours with family members you never particularly liked, getting fat on food you definitely don't like, and watching TV shows that nearly put you off the medium for life isn't bad enough.

Quite when it became an accepted truth that one should wear really weird clothes at Christmas is not entirely clear. Possibly it coincided with the rise in the horror that is the office Christmas party throughout the '80s and up to—oh lucky us—the present day. Here is an event in which people will suddenly be gripped by the desire to show how crazy and fun they are normally, beneath their PowerPoint-happy exteriors. All those across-the-floor crushes, long-term grievances, and the general repression nurtured throughout the year come to full flower in a cavernous room filled with discarded plastic cups, watery white wine, and the pulsating tune of (the now forever ruined) "Hey Ya!" Velvet is a well-beloved fabric for a woman at an office Christmas party 'cause, like, it's festive but also a bit sexy in that it makes men want to stroke you, right? No, it makes men wonder why you're dressed up like the coffee table at their in-laws'. For the male boss, a velvet waistcoat is the perfect thing for showing that he's as up for a bit of—chortle, chortle—festive fun as the next Dire Straits fan.

As for the man in a velvet suit, ask yourself this: is a '70s lounge singer really what you reckon every woman dreams of bringing home to Mum and Dad one day? You're not Sammy Davis Jr. Get over it.

Vintage

Vintage, schmintage—it's not the concept of it that bothers me, it's the snotty-faced justifications behind its recent and apparently untoppable election to the apex of the fashion pyramid.

To recap, as probably even your former geography teacher knows, vintage is the most fashionable label to wear these days. Indeed, let's ask a current issue of a typical glossy fashion magazine for their opinion: "Forget Chanel, forget Armani—everybody who's anybody is wearing vintage." And really, who can argue with such deathless prose?

Ever since people (aka Kate Moss) popularized vintage clothes about a decade ago, her followers have come up with some rum old justifications for this trend:

1. "Only vintage clothes fit my small shape." As a modern lady with a modern body built by modern foods like Crunchy Nut Cornflakes and Bacardi Breezers, I have little truck with that.
2. "They don't make clothes like they used to," which is as annoying and erroneous as saying something like "TV has really gone downhill since the 1960s."

3. "At least no one else will be wearing this dress at the party," a concern that would seem to display an impressive lack of a sense of humor.

Vintage came into fashion basically when lots of models started wearing it, models being the only species on earth that has sufficient time to trawl through racks of dead people's clothes to find the occasional nugget, the funds to buy it, and the body to make anything—even dead people's clothes—look good. And as all loyal readers of *InStyle* and *Elle* know, once a model is spotted in something, that particular garment is obviously A Good Thing. And there were, I fully concede, some rather nice pieces unearthed: Kate Moss in a smashing yellow dress; um, Kate Moss in a polka-dot dress; er, Kate in a shimmering gold minidress. And, you know, I'm sure there are plenty more to be found. But really, who has time for all that digging through piles of crap, all that rifling through jumbled clothes racks, all those cold mornings going to street markets and digging through trash bags? Whatever happened to a good old-fashioned shop where everything's labeled nicely and various sizes are available? Yes, maybe that does make me a brainwashed sheep, but you know what? I'm a brainwashed sheep with more free time on my hands for that little thing called "having a life."

Also, I'm not saying that a fair amount of modern fashion leaves something to be desired, but this is not quite the same thing as saying everything old is good. For a start, you have to ask yourself why, if this stuff is so great, has somebody given it away in the first place? I've seen a pair of beaten-up old DMs that were going for $200 because they were "early '90s originals"; I've seen tea-stained H&M tops being dubbed "original

'80s." Go on eBay and anything that is clearly a bit of old tat finds absolution in the label "vintage." What nice stuff there was in the vintage market is now priced to such hilarious levels that it somewhat undermines vintage's original image as the bohemian alternative and a good ol' blow at capitalism. And we haven't even mentioned the other joys of vintage shopping, such as being sneered at by the vendor for not recogizing that something was "an original" (truly, the only thing worse than a vintage fashion snob is a vintage-fashion-seller snob); having to listen to the seller bark on about how Kate Moss/Alexander McQueen/John Galliano get all their stuff from them (Kate Moss is the link between vintage sellers and drug dealers—every single blessed person in both of those professions claims to have had dealings with the young lady); realizing that every piece of vintage you've bought actually just makes you look like Miss Havisham and/or an extra from *Dynasty*; and having to quell the strong suspicion that you are being royally ripped off. Vintage shops often have an intriguing aversion to putting price tags on their clothes. Possibly this is because their amazing wares accrue value with every passing day. Possibly for some other reason. Who really can say?

The truth is, there is a suspicious synchronicity between the moment when vintage became fashionable and the mass market got good. I don't want to come over all Oliver Stone here, but one can't help wondering if the reason people started cooing over one-offs and overpriced 1970s dresses is because the masses were suddenly able, for the first time in quite a while, to buy decent clothes for themselves. Quick! We have to find some way to make them feel that isn't quite good enough! I know! Let's tell them that the mass market is manufactured garbage, whereas if you really want to keep it real you have to pay $1,400 for an Ossie Clark dress from Rellik! Yeah, baby—that's what I call staying grounded.

Volume, and the ironic cruelty of the oversized cut

When these balloon, pouffed, sack, or whatever-euphemism-you-prefer shapes reemerged in the early half of this century, it looked, at first, like designers had finally begun to realize that life does not stop at 98 pounds. Ah, glory be! customers cried. Clothes that one can wear when over a size 8 and not look like a sausage stuffed by an overenthusiastic factory worker! Dresses that don't crush one's ribs or collapse one's lungs! How fortunate we are!

In fact, voluminous clothes turned out to be even more fascistic about size than the tightest catsuit in Nancy Dell'Olio's wardrobe, because they depend on (dramatic, ominous cinematic close-up) contrast. Just as clothes that appear to be from Miss Havisham's wardrobe—oversized cardigans, Chanel-esque tweed jackets, pencil-skirt suits—ironically look best on young women simply because on anyone else they would look, well, old, so oversized clothes can only be worn on the very, very thin. A sacklike dress on a twiglike woman emphasizes her twigginess. But a sacklike dress on a larger woman merely looks like it's the only thing she could fit into. This is what is known as a fashion tease: you think, at last, your needs have been recognized, only then to discover that it's all for someone whose needs are already well and truly met. It's like when the gorgeous boy at school starts to hang around with you for, you think, your fabulous sense of humor and encyclopedic knowledge of '80s indie bands. But in fact, he's still getting off with the cheerleaders behind the sheds and using you for a bit of quirky cred.

The one upside to this cruel twist of fashion fate is that this rule is generally apparent only to those in the fashion world. The sharp twist in that tail is that, to most people, no one looks good in baggy clothes because, well, they're baggy. You can bandy about phrases such as "Cristóbal Balenciaga's original sack dress" and "*très* Paul Poiret" all you like, but ultimately, unless onlookers have well and truly affixed their fashion goggles upon their twitchy little noses, they will simply think you are wearing a sack, Paul Poiret be damned.

This is not to say that volume as a whole need be dismissed or that Ms. Dell'Olio had it right all along. It just needs to be used like salt, with a delicate and health-conscious pinch. So instead of a full-on sack, just wear a loose top and then, as a compromising nod to those who don't care about Balenciaga's original quasi-couture styles, narrow trousers or a similarly fitting skirt. Alternatively, you could go for a tight-bodice-style top and then a puffed-out skirt, but many women tend to favor the former approach, partly because they feel a bit daft dressing like ballerinas when they're over twenty-five (unless they are actually ballerinas, of course, in which case, fair enough) and partly because many prefer to keep the area around their stomach hidden beneath soothing folds of fabric. Thus it doesn't look like you are hiding beneath swaths of material to disguise the parts of you that you'd rather not be faced with every hour of the livelong day and cheekily flaunting your best assets (even if that is exactly what you're doing), but rather that you're being ever so insouciantly modest and, by heavens, if that is how good her legs are, imagine what she has going on beneath that smock top! And returning to the earlier example of geriatric chic, it ultimately comes down to clever contrast: a Chanel-style jacket with a pair of jeans—good; a Chanel-style jacket with a Chanel-style tweed skirt—how many will be joining you for lunch at Le Caprice, Lady von '80s Throwback?

An interesting combination of these rules was proffered to the masses by a, thankfully, short-lived trend masterminded by celebrity stylist Rachel Zoe. Between 2005 and 2006, Zoe was the woman behind the curtain, controlling the unexpected fashion idolatry of Nicole Richie, Lindsay Lohan, and other such cultural luminaries with her coining of a trend, brilliantly dubbed by *Tatler* "The Dead Socialite Look." This trend, as the name suggests, was inspired by socialites from the past such as Nan Kempner, Babe Paley, and Slim Aarons—Ladies Who Didn't Lunch and would never knowingly mix with NQOCD (Not Quite Our Class, Darling). Charming women, one and all; thank heavens we continue to celebrate their legacy. Anyway, this look involved lots of old-ladyish tweeds, original vintage voluminous caftans, and billowing smock tops, all of which worked wonders to emphasize Richie's skinniness and wealth but on anyone over 98 pounds who couldn't afford the Pucci originals, it only made them look like Elizabeth Taylor, the Fortensky years. Thus, it managed to be both the most size-ist and class-ist trend yet coined, and for that alone Zoe's sudden if brief position as the most influential stylist of her time is well deserved.

Yoga, detoxes, and other euphemisms for exercise and diets

Even the most adamant defenders of fashion will concede that, when it comes to women's bodies in this business, thin is always more desirable than fat. However, somewhere between the late '80s and the mid-'90s, the words "diet" and "exercise" started to chime in a very off-key way. They just sounded, well, a little anachronistic—tacky, even. Which is odd, because certainly being thin had not become either of those things: if anything, the bar was being set still higher, or lower, or whatever, as the fashion ideal shifted from Cindy Crawford playing volleyball in a swimsuit to Kate Moss looking mopey in a tank top and panties in what appeared to be a crack den. So if it wasn't the goal, it must have been the methods that were tarnishing. *Et voilà,* the emergence of detoxing and yoga, which are, respectively, morally superior dieting and stretching with an added dose of self-obsession.

Once, detoxing and yoga were the embarrassing province of milky-faced, stringy-haired hippies, who played wind chimes and had distasteful sex involving chants in praise of the power of the uterus. Now, however, they were being celebrated by the most desirable sort (i.e., models, actresses, and the wealthy).

Other euphemisms that emerged included:

1. Looking after oneself
2. Going on a retreat
3. Getting healthy

This happened, in part, because of the growing concern in the media over the connection between the open-mouthed, slavering veneration of thinness and eating disorders; fashionable sorts had to find code words for their pursuit of visible bones. Pre-1996, yoga and detoxing were about separating oneself from shallow materialism, so there is something very pleasing about their being adopted as the path to that well-known spiritual state, having a flat stomach.

Dieting and aerobics fell victim to their own success, the classic casualties of market saturation. Dieting took on the flavor of daytime-TV-watching housewives, of coverline promises on weekly women's magazines, and buckets of strawberry-flavored meal-replacement powder sold in drugstores. In other words, anyone could diet. Well, what's the point of that, then? It was all right in the '80s when diet and exercise brought to mind cool aerobics instructors in sexy leotards and high-flying businessmen taking power showers. But it was definitely not all right when it became about middle-aged ladies doing leg lifts in pastel leotards on the covers of books sold in supermarkets. And if the value of thinness, like that of being blond, lies in its relative exclusivity, then it is VERY ANNOYING to see the great unwashed jumping on the same bandwagon.

Furthermore, admitting that you diet and exercise proves that you have to work at being thin. This is simply unacceptable. In addition to its previous association of laziness and gluttony, fat is now, thanks to the food fascists, a signifier of class—lower, that is—the kind of yob who sits on the sofa watching *All My Children* while eating a bag of Fritos instead of dashing about town between an acupunturist and dinner with Sienna and Keira while snacking on an organic papaya. Thus, to admit that you have to make an effort to keep thin suggests that you are a faker, a cuckoo in the nest of glamorous upper-middle-class acceptability.

And speaking of class concerns, let us not forget that it is much more expensive to detox than to diet; a bunch of organic, ethically grown and harvested-by-happy-workers cherries being a damn sight more costly than a tub of Slim-Fast. Even though one could easily lose weight by shopping at a cheap supermarket, a fridge full of Key Food products, even if they include skim milk, fruit, and water, is definitely less with-it than a cupboard of Whole Foods' own brand. The latter also suggests that, you know, you care about what you put into your body, that you know about carcinogens, pesticides, and genetic modification, whereas anyone who shops elsewhere is an uneducated, *Enquirer*-reading dullard. As with the fuss and exclusivity of vintage shopping, organic market shopping requires more time and money than just going down to the supermarket. Thus, a person who does so must (a) not have a very demanding job and, nonetheless (b) a steady flow of cash.

On a vaguely more positive note, all this detoxing and all those yoga-class waiting lists are an endearing verification of our own undeniable, unfightable, inherent laziness. It feels less self-deluding to tell yourself that you are detoxing than it does to stop eating chocolate for a week. Similarly, yoga, while potentially quite strenuous if you want to look like Madonna, is definitely less of a hellish prospect than an aerobics class. Thus, they are an optimal means to trick ourselves into being thin, as though we'll wake up one morning and find ourselves with the lithe, lean bodies of seventeen-year-olds purely from eating organic fruit 'n' nut bars and doing cat poses for a month.

Really, it's very sweet and childlike. Here we are, all puffed up with pride about our medical advances, our knowledge about the world's origins, busily booking flights to the moon, yet we still think buying a $7.95 bottle of aloe vera juice will somehow make us morally superior and painlessly thin, or that wearing something with "skinny" in the name will endow us with that very quality, and that a bit of cheap dark plastic propped in front of our eyes will convince the world that we are very, very cool. To quote that well-known fashion commentator Tiny Tim (have you seen his skinny legs? Like, beyond fabulous), God bless us, every one.

Printed in the United States
by Baker & Taylor Publisher Services